I would like to dedicate this book to my son Winter Wolfe. He is the weight missing from my arms, he is the occupier of my heart, he is the love that lifts my spirits.

I would like to dedicate this book to Áron Matzon. His life inspired his mother to draw the most beautiful illustrations. Without him, this would be a book of many words but not a single picture. He connected two mothers and countless others.

I would like to dedicate this book to every single spark of life that has left this world so swiftly but never without meaning. Teeny tiny lives, monumental love.

Throughout this book I have described babies that have died as 'lost babies'. It took a long time to settle on an appropriate phrase. Of course, we know that we do not really 'lose' a baby. They are not a set of keys or a handheld diary. They are not misplaced. We were not lackadaisical with their life. We know all too well that there will be no *finding* them. Lost baby, sleeping baby, angel baby, forever baby, whatever term we use, really we know they are simply a *loved* baby. For clarity, I made the decision to choose one phrase throughout the book, but if you wish you can choose to mentally change that as you read, to any name that will bring you the most comfort.

CONTENTS

HERE
& GONE

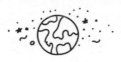

The loss of a baby – there is nothing else quite like it. A truly devastating and monumentally painful tragedy that alters your every notion of reality. Whether during a cherished pregnancy or after a baby is brought home and loved, when your baby dies your future is rewritten in an instant.

A baby's death is the polar opposite of new life. And so you take your first steps into the world of loss – in a cave with a flashlight, searching for hope and guidance.

When we lose our baby we are left crushed and bewildered. A thief has crept into our brightest dreams and darkened them, stealing not only a little beating life, but the future we had planned together. The unfathomable question rests heavy on our shoulders: *How can something that has only just begun end so swiftly?* The reality of life ceasing so abruptly before a deserving chance is so far out of the order of life that we are left blindsided and swept out to sea. There is both a sense of disconnection when we just simply cannot comprehend the magnitude of what has happened and a sense of having lost everything at once, a numb yet undeniable pain.

The circumstances of our loss can differ vastly. Missed miscarriage, when a baby is lost without any physical symptoms, a baby born silent but perfect, an infant birthed and buried as fast as the sun rose and set, a pregnancy that gently held the tiniest of sparks, a child who was taken home healthy and plucked so suddenly from our grip, a babe we willed through illness but who sadly could not stay.

My personal journey into the world of baby loss began with the loss of my son. I became pregnant quickly, and I had a gentle and healthy pregnancy experience. There were no complications expected and I had no real understanding of loss. After a natural and fairly uneventful labour, our little boy Winter Wolfe was delivered and placed onto my chest. We held him close, so full of newborn awe that we didn't even manage a photograph before he suddenly stopped breathing and was whisked away to be resuscitated. At one day old, our baby could not be saved. We held him in our arms and felt his heart drum its last little beat. I became a bereaved mother, forever loving and missing my Winter. And our journey to a living baby was yet to throw more obstacles and pain, as two early miscarriages left us further heartbroken.

In circumstances that can be so drastically varied, it is difficult to encapsulate those early days of loss and be thoroughly inclusive, but there are, among the variations, moments shared by many. If you had the great fortune of physically meeting your baby for the first time after death or in the brief moments before, you will have discovered it is simultaneously a painful and beautiful event. Among the brutal devastation of an all too early death, we find there is a steely and unwavering pleasure in meeting our baby. Holding them is our opportunity to study their face, to feel their weight, to touch their skin, simple pleasures that are all too soon to be denied. The need to kiss and cuddle your baby is the most natural feeling for a new mother.

There is a need to document as much as possible, yet in those early confusing moments you may not have fully known what you wanted to photograph, or what memories you wanted to create. It is such an intense moment to be so dramatically tossed into. You could only look to those around you for guidance and trust to follow your own motherly instincts. There is the realisation that this is all the memories you will make, your time together is limited to this very moment. It is a heavy weight to carry, time has never before felt so precious and fleeting. And no matter how we spend that time, no matter how long we have, it will never be enough. What is important is the knowledge that in that moment, that immensely difficult and intense moment, you did all that you could.

Further down the line, as you look back, you will inevitably play that moment out and wish there were things you had done differently. Regrets will rise, perhaps realisations of missed opportunity within that short time you had.

Even if you had physically carried your baby to the moon and back to show them the endless magnitude of your love, you would still sit today wishing, If only we had ...

Among the endless circumstances, there are situations where families choose not to see their baby after death. The opportunity to hold their physical appearance within the safe and loving realms of immaculate imagination is an opportunity too prized to pass. The knowledge that your baby is perfect in every which way needs no validation from the naked eye.

Regardless of meeting, you still hold bounds of love and pride alongside your baby's memory, the two come together like a feather and a wing. The tragic circumstances are at some point null and void – you are simply a proud mother to a baby, here or gone, dead or alive. When you lose your baby you face a wealth of emotions, and although these may include misplaced feelings of guilt and failure, you also do not stop feeling love, and you do not stop feeling pride.

In the instances where your baby has been cared for before they died, whether premature or unwell, within the hospital or apparently healthy at home, you will have established a routine of looking after them. As with any newborn baby, your lives have met exceptional change in what is famously a sleep-deprived and non-stop experience. Your baby's death creates not only an instant loss physically and emotionally, but also the abrupt end to a constant familiar routine. The sudden halt is colossal and flattening, and leaves an immense emptiness within day-to-day life. Time suddenly seems plentiful and suffocating as the time you spent caring for your baby is left unfilled.

If you lost your baby in late pregnancy or after birth, there is a good chance that in the aftermath you were confronted with a home bustling with baby preparations or items used and touched by your baby. Babies lost much earlier, and therefore before the chance for preparation arose, will still have memories attached to objects around the home. In the days and weeks that follow, you may choose to keep your preparations as they are, finding some solace in the love you lavished on your baby, perhaps before you even met them. A nursery that remains untouched or used so very briefly is both beyond precious and inherently painful. The dish we cooked when we discovered we were pregnant, the outfit we first noticed a tiny bump in. Other times you may feel that the stark emptiness is too palpable and make the decision to pack away some items. While we kept our son's nursery as it was right up until we moved house, the vast and obvious lack of a baby in the Moses basket proved too difficult and I gifted it to a charity shop.

As with any grief journey, there is never a right or wrong. With the great gift of hindsight, however, I tentatively suggest that you keep hold of some items, even if you initially feel they are too painful to keep. Maybe you can pass them on to family to store for you, or pack them lovingly into the loft. So many loss mothers, myself included, wish they had kept some items for their future babies, as a way of connecting siblings beyond physical presence – an idea that, in the early throes of loss, can feel entirely unimaginable.

Our baby's death can all happen so quickly, in such a small time frame in our long stretch of life, that it can feel as though it were all a dream.

In these early moments, as with any loss journey, everyone reacts and grieves so differently it is impossible to explore all the different emotions we may encounter. Some grieve heavily in the immediate aftermath, the realisation of the permanence of death is instant and consuming. Others are left too numbed by shock to fully take stock of all that their loss truly means. I know many, many fellow loss friends who sought solace in the comfort of their own home, and mostly in their bed, and perhaps this is you too. It's as though you have your own little safety den, where you can be certain not to bump into people and have to explain; a place where you can lick your wounds and try to comprehend the enormity of your new circumstance. Certainly even now, when feeling particularly daunted by grief, I retreat to bed.

If your bump was visible or you had the honour of announcing your news, then suddenly regular social and daily pit stops can become a source of much anxiety as you wonder how many times you will have to revisit the beautiful but still freshly painful story of your baby. Wondering who you will meet and who will notice your bump has disappeared. Who will exclaim 'You've had the baby!' and who will ask the details. Answering those questions and explaining the less than ideal circumstance rarely comes easily to loss mothers. Taking some time to role play in the safety of your own home, mastering the response you are most comfortable with, is a good idea.

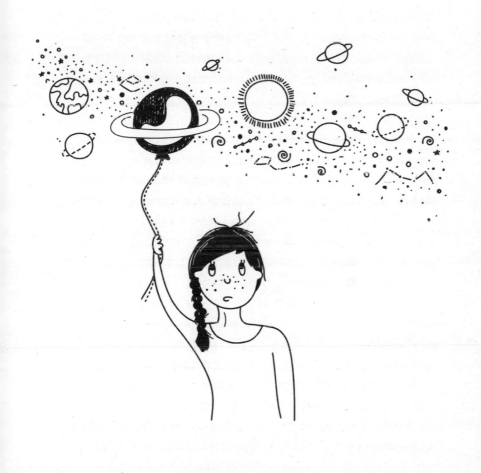

With earlier miscarriage – perhaps robbed of the chance even to announce your happy news – the initial anxiety is still palpable as you step out into the world, a changed person harvesting an unseen loss. You may be faced with other difficult questions, 'When do you plan to start a family?' There will be many moments where you are faced with such daunting questions, and so early on in loss they will leave you feeling vulnerable and lost. Over time and with practice your replies will become more sturdy and confident.

Sharing news of our loss with others is a huge source of anxiety. If you simply cannot find the words yourself, or the task feels far too intense, you can call on friends and family to do this in your place. There is also the opportunity to embrace social media as a way of continuing your baby's journey. It's a choice you can make, neither right nor wrong, and much of that depends on just how active you were online in the lead up to your baby's life and death.

Dean and I chose to share news of our son's death pretty much immediately, alongside a small selection of photographs. I found it a good decision for us. Having documented the pregnancy I knew my friends and family were expecting news of his birth at any moment, and I was afraid of having to explain over and over why my bump had gone but my arms were not full. Writing a status sharing our news saved us from many difficult future interactions – so many people informed in one swift click of the laptop.

I did the same when I miscarried, despite not even having shared news of my pregnancy. While some who do not understand this journey may consider this to be 'over-sharing', anyone who experiences the loneliness of miscarriage will know there is an unmet need for this subject to be spoken about openly. It is such a hushed 'private' trauma that we are often left quietly seeking solace and understanding in closed forums and sites dedicated solely to such loss. If anyone wondered why I chose to share such personal experiences, I reminded them that my babies were loved, no matter how brief their life; they are important to me, they were the beginning of an alternative future that will now never materialise and their existence warranted marking. When I shared news of my miscarriages, it was as though I was peeking from under a blanket, one eye open, wondering, *Is anyone else out there?* And there was, lots of people, peeking back out at me, reaching out to hold my hand. So I threw off the blanket and stretched. I wasn't alone, we are not alone.

As with many brief lives, my son's birth announcement also carried the news of his death. And I shared the news of my son because I wanted to. Like any other new mother I wanted to announce my creation to the world. One of my most poignant memories from those early days of grief was the desire to show off my baby. I had spent so long waiting for him, planning his announcement and wondering what he would look like. When he died, I still wanted the world to see him but I was afraid to show him off. His face was blanketed in tubes and wires, his lips were darkened and his skin was losing colour. But I didn't see that.

Mothers see past the blemishes left behind by death. They don't see a dead baby, they see a loved, wanted, perfect baby.

You may choose to keep your baby private, perhaps you feel their photos are too precious to share, and of course that is always your own choice and one you should feel confident to make. Alternatively, if you decide to share then you can take that leap with the knowledge that you are as justified as a mother with a living baby. You are not only allowing the world to see the beauty of your creation, but you are opening the eyes of those around you to the realisation that not all baby's come home and grow into adults – you are reminding them how prized their own babies are.

If you face resistance then you can take the opportunity to gently educate with your decision. I was faced with this very dilemma myself when a friend questioned very publicly why anyone would share images of a baby that has died. I was deeply, deeply hurt. The very idea that my son was offensive in some way and should be hidden away so shamefully hurt like hell. So I spoke out. We don't need to shame those who are so misguided and confused that they cannot understand our choices, we simply need to explain our decision with the pride and love we hold for our baby. It goes without saying that bereaved families should not have to face such barriers, and yet we do, still. If you want to show off your baby, do it.

I would like to begin this book with not only the recognition of our deep-felt pain, but also with the offering of hope. We all know the hurt that ravages us after loss, we all know the dark places that we are pulled to, and as mothers we also know the wonderful love our baby's presence brought with them.

You hurt because you loved, you will continue to hurt because you will continue to love. When we peel away the loss, the death, the tears, the pain, when we rewind from the tragedy that stole our dreams, when we bring ourselves to the very beginning point of this fretful path, the initial feeling is that of love. Love for your baby, love for the future you planned together. Love really is the dominating emotion, it was the catalyst of your journey, it was the very first domino to fall. As your journey continues, your grief – although never-ending – becomes familiar and more manageable in your day-to-day life.

Anger, jealousy, resentment, the cascade of emotions is intense – life after baby loss is hard. But each and every time it comes back to love, the loudest emotion.

Trust from here on in that this love will prevail, it will keep you afloat. You will find ways to celebrate and include your baby, you will make it through this chapter of life not just surviving, but thriving, always with your baby held close in your heart. Dark days are ahead of you, and so are lighter ones. It's a mixed bag – an immeasurable loss has been thrust upon you, and over time you will discover that where there is deep loss, there is also deep gain. Our babies simply cannot exist without leaving behind something great, and although nothing can ever make up for the treachery of a little life stolen, they are deserving of warm thoughts and a smile at their memory. And it will come, if not in this instant, with time. Whether we laugh fondly at their belly kicks and rolls, their fat feet and the nose inherited from Uncle Fred, or the ridiculous cravings their pregnancy brought with them, over time, this lighter energy will emerge. Keep hope.

And so here is a gentle summary of suggestions when you are so fresh in the face of loss:

❋ Be kind to yourself. Allow grief, allow yourself to hurt. Do not inflict self-judgement on your emotions, simply feel.

❋ Try to look back at your time with your baby with as few regrets as possible. Each moment you carried them was special, any time you had together was unique and cannot ever be replicated *or replaced*. Those moments are yours forever.

❋ Ask friends and family to share your news if you feel it is too difficult. Keep your baby private if you wish to and hold them tightly in your heart.

❋ Or share the news yourself and your baby's photographs if you feel this is right for you. Whatever you choose is personal and right for your journey.

❋ If it is too painful to see them each day, arrange for any baby preparations to be stored lovingly away. Keep them out if they are a warm reminder of your baby's life.

❋ Remember that your baby's existence was ignited by love, and that love is the very catalyst for all you are about to experience. Hold on to that love.

HOPE &
HEARTBREAK

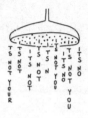

Baby loss comes in many forms – miscarriage, stillbirth or neonatal death. Sometimes the baby is sick and being cared for, other times a healthy baby dies suddenly at home. The experiences differ greatly, but the foundation of the suffering is much the same. When a baby is lost, at whatever age and in whatever circumstance, there is pain and heartbreak left for the bereaved. As I touched on in the previous chapter, while all loss is still surrounded in a (slowly lifting) taboo, miscarriage can feel particularly isolating and hushed. The nature of losing your baby before they were announced to the world, or before a bump provided visible evidence of their life, is an experience that can leave us feeling particularly abandoned.

Miscarriage is a thoroughly lonely experience. When my son died at full term and one day old, I had photographs and physical mementos, such as a lock of hair and a footprint. People around me had followed our pregnancy journey, they knew we were expecting a baby and they joined in with our excitement and anticipation, and therefore it was possible for them to join in with our grief and heartbreak when he died so suddenly. I was visibly pregnant, he had visibly died. But my experience with my early losses was very different. Miscarriages are concealed to the outside world, they feel private, secretive, and so our grief mirrors that. Whereas a baby born later in pregnancy can be celebrated and adored, the brief life of a womb baby feels so much more difficult to speak about publicly. Without an opportunity to share our happy news we are denied the opportunity to share our sadness. Miscarriage is as if we are a victim of a robbery on a desert island. No witnesses to the crime, no one to arrest, no evidence to the wider world of our suffering. It all happened *in us*, and we feel separated from the world.

One day we are pregnant, the next we are not. One day walking the earth with another little life in our womb, the next we are just one single person. And to the eyes of those around us, nothing changed, we remained the same; the world and its inhabitants are none the wiser.

Our loneliness comes not only from the invisibility of our loss, but also the misunderstandings of how deep that loss runs. I experienced a huge inner battle to keep my equilibrium as I slipped into the torrid confusion and stigma that society appears to blanket upon miscarriage. Comments like 'It's not even a real baby yet' whirled around in my head. At what point is it a real baby? When it has a heartbeat? Eyes? Limbs? Consciousness? A soul? It is impossible to define.

For many of us it is a real baby the moment we see the positive test, because that is the moment a wistful dream has become a sturdy reality. It is a real baby because it has a real chance at a future, a real place in our imagination, a real tiny little spark that would, without tragedy, grow into a real human. The moment we see that positive test we work out our due date, how old they will be at Christmas time, wonder if we will grow a boy or a girl. When we lose our baby, all our hopeful dreams are snatched from us like a thief stealing our future.

Once you're pregnant you begin a whole new journey, life darts off into another exciting direction, there is no feat greater and more meaningful than placing a fresh life on earth. Miscarriage is the cruel traitor that plucks us from the joyful path and abandons us back to our old journey. We are left feeling hollow and hopeless, so much excitement and joy replaced with a shattered reality.

There is no greater word to describe the feeling than 'empty', both physically and emotionally empty. We have not just lost our pregnancy, we have lost our *baby*, our *chance* at a baby, our *future* with a baby. Our calendar, once filled so excitedly with dates and plans, now appears scattered and painfully blank, and we are left to carry on. And while your life resumes you are forever changed by your new-found motherhood and the big 'what if' that your tiny womb baby left behind. Everything you hoped for, all that you had mentally and emotionally set out in front of you, swiped away without trace.

So how can we help to keep this loneliness at bay?

The first thing we can do is find others who share in our heartbreak. Those who understand the pain, those we can connect with and find friendly solace in.

It turns out that miscarriage is alarmingly common. Once it happened to me it seemed as though everyone I spoke to had suffered a similar fate. I wondered why no one had ever told me. It was as if there was a secret club with endless members, but you only knew about it when you were qualified to join by experience. I shared my personal story and watched as my virtual and real-life friends raised their hands and whispered, 'Me too.'

Such is the expectation for miscarriage to be private and hushed that I was unaware of even those close to me who had lost in such a similar way. And with this discovery I was warmly exposed to a new-found sisterhood. Online too, there is an immense community readily available to support you through your loss. As well as the list provided in the back of this book, I can wholeheartedly recommend searching the #babyloss and #miscarriage hashtags on both Instagram and Twitter, where there is an endless sea of fellow miscarriage mothers.

The next thing you can do to ease that lonesome feeling is to bravely tell those around you just why you are hurting so deeply. It can prove nerve-racking. When talking about miscarriage it can feel as though you are baring a very intimate moment. The term 'mis-carriage' insinuates that

we, the owner of the womb, simply misplaced something.
It certainly does nothing to aid the relief of shame. How
dastardly of us to misplace something so important — were
we not careful enough? Of course this is not true at all, but
with such deeply ingrained emotions it can feel impossible
to convince ourselves otherwise. And it can be this feeling of
'not being good enough' that holds us back from speaking out.
We don't want to bare our souls and we don't want the silent
judgement we expect in return. But if you can find your voice,
no matter how quiet and wobbly, then speaking out is what
you can do. You can understand why those around you are
left dumbfounded and possibly ignorant to your pain, and you
can gently explain – lifting the fog of silence, and smoothing
out the clumsy comfort that is offered.

It can be difficult even for a pregnant mother to envisage
her unborn baby. We may see the lines on the test and we
may have the opportunity to analyse the tiny beginnings on a
grainy scan, and we may understand in our motherly wisdom
that life has already long begun in our womb, but *believing* it
can be a whole other obstacle. Even if we progress far enough
in pregnancy to carry an enormous bump and feel punches
and rolls, we still walk around never really believing that
there is an actual life inside it. And if it is hard for us to grasp
the miracle of a babe in our own belly, then for others around
us it could be even trickier. This is the hurdle when grieving
a miscarriage, when even our loved ones may not fully
understand the pain that comes with the loss of such tiny life.
And so you can say, 'It hurts. For me it was real, my baby is
important to me and I am grieving for that loss.'

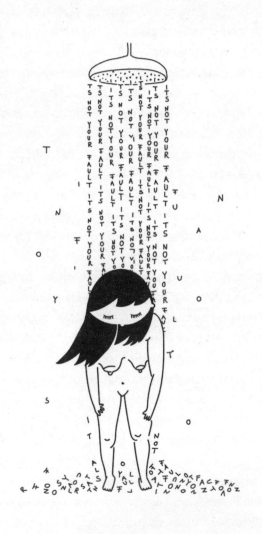

You must allow yourself the honour of grieving. I've spoken to so many mothers who have miscarried who feel undeserving of their right to grieve because they have been told 'It could have been worse … baby could have been born and died', etc. But honestly, what is worse? Miscarriage, infertility, stillbirth, neonatal death. That's a bloody painful line-up and there is no scorecard. A mother without her baby is a mother without her baby, regardless of the circumstances leading up to it. If we long to be a mother and we are left empty handed, or with a face forever missing from our family photographs, then we share much the same pain as other mothers who find themselves without their child. It's true that I couldn't compare the loss of my one-day-old son to my miscarriages, but it's also true that I couldn't compare either of my miscarriages to each other, and nor could I compare the loss of my son to the loss of someone else's son, or my own experience of miscarriage to someone else's experience of miscarriage.

Competitive grief and trying to figure out who has the worst scenario is a weird reality of life after loss, but given thought we can realise it is ultimately a waste of time and much-needed energy. Suffering is suffering, pain is pain, loss is loss. Grief is complex, every single person mourns differently and there are a million different events that can lead up to a loss. Some may argue that one is worse than the other, but I think we can all agree that when a baby dies, no one wins. Whether that baby was four womb days old or four earth days old, no baby is no baby.

Gestation and circumstance are tragic embellishments –
any pregnancy, or wish for pregnancy, that ends without a
baby at home is never the 'better situation'. Comparison of
pain is futile.

A spark of life extinguished was still a L I F E once.
Miscarriage hurts, it is a loss and it must be recognised as
such. Mothers who gained their title with a positive test only
to lose their baby the very next day, and mothers birthing
their tiny babies with hands and feet as small as a bird's
footprint in the snow. The lines of miscarriage and stillbirth
are blurred, and the official title is ultimately irrelevant.
Dr Seuss wrote, 'A person's a person, no matter how small'
and there is nothing but truth in that.

I once read somewhere, rather offensively, that a
miscarriage is 'just like having a period'. Except it's not, it's
not at all like that. A period is part of your body's natural
cycle, and even that is difficult enough to experience
when you are trying so desperately to have a baby. But a
miscarriage, no matter how early on in pregnancy, is not only
physically much more than a period, it is emotionally much
deeper than that. It is the beginning of a life that your body
can no longer hold on to, it is the start of something special
that ended far too soon. And so you must allow yourself time
to grieve.

Remove any inner burden that suggests you are not
entitled to hurt; we are all entitled to hurt. As the saying
goes, you can close your eyes to what you do not want to

see, but you cannot close your heart to what you do not want to feel.

There are the endless questions. The confusing reality that our wombs can both harvest life and cradle death. It all seems so abrupt, a life beginning that suddenly just stopped. When I miscarried I spent a lot of time trying to figure out why. I had had one pregnancy that was as problem-free as possible but ended with the death of my one-day-old son, followed by two early losses. My miscarriages felt like salt in the wound, the final hurrah of what I imagined would be a childless future. I was sent for some basic testing, but was left with no explanation greater than, 'It is just one of those things'.

So often miscarriage is left with question marks, and the not knowing is so disorienting. We feel completely helpless. You are left questioning everything. *Was it something I ate or a movement I made?* The desperation to just know with confident certainty the reason for the loss is overwhelming. We *need* to know so that we can avoid the same fate again and again, we *need* to assure ourselves that any future pregnancies will be safe. And yet it is often an impossible need to fulfil. Research into miscarriage is still, sadly, underfunded, undervalued and in its infancy, and all too often mothers are left to pick up the pieces and simply wish for the best in future pregnancies.

But if we feel our care is not taken seriously or we are suffering from repeated loss, then we can take our voices with us to the doctors, we can *insist* on more testing. We can empower ourselves with knowledge. Tommy's, the baby charity, are leading the way with their research and expertise into baby loss, and their website offers a wealth of additional information and support around miscarriage. It is not 'just one of those things', it is a painful loss, it deserves attention and you deserve at least the opportunity to find out why.

And so when experiencing a loss through miscarriage you can:

❋ Seek out others who share your experience, in real life and online.
❋ Explain to those around you the pain you feel and why.
❋ Allow yourself to grieve; miscarriage is a valid and painful loss.
❋ Voice your concerns to healthcare professionals and seek answers.
❋ Visit Tommy's website for a great depth of miscarriage information.

LIFE GOES ON

After the initial blow of your loss, you face an array
of mismatched emotions, in varying orders, flows and
intensities. Anger, jealousy, deep sadness, pride and even
bittersweet happiness – you are tossed from one to the next
with little respite. And alongside this new emotional tornado
you discover that life goes on, that the dishwasher still needs
emptying, the food shop still need doing, the bills still need
paying. You feel grief settle into your bones; you become
accustomed to the daily grind of life with the stagnant feeling
that something is missing, that your life should be so different
to the experience now laid out in front of you. That your bump
should be growing, your baby should be breathing.

*You exist simultaneously within two worlds; the world
of your loss and the 'real' world.*

And now you are left feeling fragile with uncertainty, and
a blank chapter you are yet to embrace. Your life has always
and forever been divided into a before and after, before your
baby existed where you felt anchored and in control, and the

after where your peace has been sabotaged. In the beginning you may have been carried by the deep love you hold for your baby, the pride and the bereft excitement to meet them regardless of circumstance. The early days may have been numbing for you, your situation changed so hastily that it takes time for your heart to catch up with the truth.

After our son died, I distinctly remember a feeling of 'still waiting'. Nine long months for his arrival, here and gone in a single day. The drawn-out lead-up of pregnancy offset the shutter speed of his lifetime. His life in the outside world was always meant to be longer than his life spent in my womb; the balance had become so topsy-turvy that half of me remained convinced we were still awaiting his arrival and at times doubting if I ever really met him at all.

When I miscarried there was a similar feeling. Continuing through life and passively accepting its daily offerings, but always the lost pregnancy playing out in the background. Living through a reflection and at the mercy of our own imagination, the pregnancy does not physically continue but we silently hit the milestones: *I would be six months pregnant now, I would be having my scan now, I would be due now, the baby would be two months old now* ... An invisible child carried with us through our whole life.

We want to stay forever connected to our baby, we always wish to hold them just once, or once more, and our deep desire to stay close to them can leave us with a strong aversion to the passing of time. Occasions that will never be fulfilled, monthly anniversaries rolling by, and as the first year passes time seems to gather speed – like string rolling down a hill that we are left chasing – and we are desperate to catch it and pause long enough to breathe and reflect. Even two-and-a-half years after my son died, and two years on from my first miscarriage, I still look back at those days with only foggy reflection and wonder if it all really happened. I've never managed to catch the string.

When you lose a baby it is so difficult to be present in the here and now. Whether a miscarriage, stillbirth or a baby that lives briefly out of womb, the enormity of the situation and the abruptness of the loss can understandably take time to truly sink in. We go through the motions, we continue to live, the memory of our baby is forever present, but every now and then we are struck with the brutal reality. A pregnant lady at the petrol station, a baby in a pram at the park, tiny booties in the shop window, nappies at the supermarket. These are the moments when you are thrown back into your grief, when you are confronted with all that you have lost.

Be gentle, be patient with your heart. Allow yourself the moments of pain. There is no way you should feel at any time in this journey, only how you do feel.

Those around you may be continually supportive, or they may not. As time rolls on, you may find that for others around you the 'novelty' (for want of a better word) wears thin. The weight of misled Western expectation leaves us feeling as though we should be moving on, we should be healing by now. People we have held close may peel themselves away from the scene of devastation, frightened or too inept to face dealing with the ongoing nature of grief. Even those who are devoting their time and energy to you may struggle to understand the scope of loss you face and its everlasting impact.

Your baby may have existed physically only very briefly, but you have lost a lifetime of memories with them, and it can feel so difficult to communicate your loss with the impact it deserves. What we want to say is that we didn't just lose our baby in that instant, but we lost them as part of our life forever. Other people who are not experienced in the loss of a baby may accuse the grieving of living in the past or clinging on to something long gone, but while the loss of your baby may be several months or years ago to them, to you it is *every day*. You lost the first smile, first giggle, first steps. You lost the sticky handprints on the glass window, the tears at a grazed knee and the Mother's Day gift made from yogurt pots. You lost the graduation, the wedding, the grandchildren.

Your loss is not a flash in the pan, it is not a short-lived event, it is continuous and never-ending.

You watch as the world moves on around you and you are frozen in a moment. You wonder how others dare to find joy when you feel so swamped in suffering. The past continues to be present. Bereaved families wake up every single morning and go to bed every night with the memory of their baby and the hole their loss has left behind.

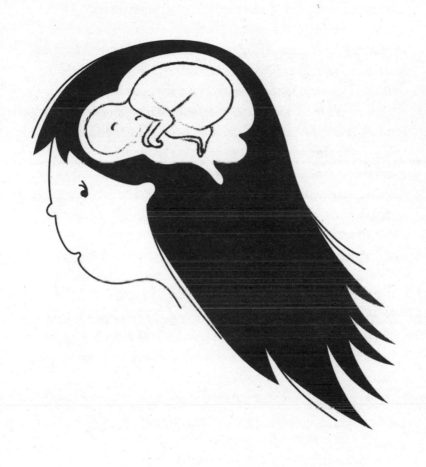

YOU ARE ALWAYS ON MY MIND.

If anyone wonders why I still talk about my son, my question to them is, 'When do you plan to stop talking about your children?' Living or not, no matter how brief their life, your baby remains part of your life forever. You can always be kind to yourself, safe in the knowledge that feeling as though you are stuck in the moments with your baby is OK – it's normal, it's natural. It is no different from holding on to the memory of a family celebration or a fond childhood moment. Revisiting that memory over and over is our way of keeping it fresh. Your mind is so powerful, so much of your baby's life exists only within your own memory, within a little glass box that is equal parts fragile and sturdy. Your memory is your most precious keepsake.

There are many instances within the world of baby loss where the bereaved are kept at such arm's length that they are left feeling as though their loss is contagious. There are so many stories of old friends crossing the road to avoid an awkward conversation, or simply failing to call or text. We can be left feeling as though people wouldn't want to spend time with us simply due to our loss, as though we are a black cloud or that our 'bad luck' will rub off onto them. It's important to remember that you are in charge of your own thoughts and actions, but not of others'. At a time when we are left so desolate in the aftermath of baby loss, relieve yourself of the pressures of others' actions and expectations. Seek out those who understand and make effort to alleviate your pain. Keep the better experiences at the forefront of your mind and use bad experiences as motivation to gently educate and change the unrealistic expectations of baby loss.

Hold close those who reach out, those who try. Perhaps their words may not always be the comfort you were hoping for, but when heartfelt effort is made, we can dismiss the delivery and focus on the intention.

You may begin to develop some rituals and find new connections to your baby. Maybe a bird, a symbol, a colour or a flower that brings you close to them. Snowflakes and wolves remind me of my son Winter, and coconuts remind me of a baby I miscarried. It can be as obscure as you want, and no doubt there will be something you have in mind already. Sharing this image with loved ones and saying 'this is how I remember my baby' gives them an opportunity to join in your remembrance. When they see that plant or animal or letter or fruit, your baby will be projected to the forefront of their mind. If you are happily willing, they may share those moments with you, and you will be reminded that your baby lives on in the memory of others too.

Returning to work can be a huge hurdle post loss. It's difficult to explain to those without the experience of losing their baby the magnitude of such a milestone. Returning to work signifies the end of your time off, time that should have been continuing your pregnancy or raising a baby. It is as though you are faced with the reality that life must return to how it was before your loss, a reality that we do not want to accept. Returning feels like another defeat. Your job can suddenly become incredibly difficult, your mind still muddled and not at all able to focus on much else other than the trauma you have experienced.

The nature of your work can suddenly become a challenge. Working with babies or young children, or within a workplace with pregnant colleagues, can transform what was once a job we loved to something much more complex. Working in a place which ticked both of these boxes, I had to re-evaluate my emotional approach. I decided early on that while being surrounded by young ones could easily inject a plethora of negative triggers, I would instead focus on caring for them how I wished I could care for my own child. In this sense I felt as though I was continuing to honour my son, offering up the love I had for him to others who needed it.

With an early loss, pre-bump and pre-announcement, taking time off and allowing yourself space to reflect can feel daunting, but don't forget that you are entitled to grieve regardless of how early on you lose your baby, and you are hurting just as anyone hurts when they miscarry. When the pregnancy is not yet public knowledge and you would like to keep the loss discreet, then seek out a colleague you have connection with and can confide in privately, someone who can 'have your back' in moments when you need headspace at work. Invite them over for tea or coffee and talk to them, not only about what has happened, but the magnitude of pain it causes, early days or not.

With any loss it is almost impossible to put all your thoughts and emotions to one side and centre yourself entirely in work. I know that I felt constantly fatigued yet unable to sleep, and while I chose to return and wanted desperately to be out of the house and busy around familiar friends, I spent much of my time there with a churning stomach and an absent mind. It is impossible to say how each person who reads this will feel about their return to work, but there is a universal feeling in the baby loss world of it being a significant marker along the loss journey, and your employer's response can either encourage your healing or send you plummeting. If it is possible, I suggest you arrange a meeting at your workplace where you can vocalise your worries and direct your colleagues to sites and information that could help them to understand how you are feeling.

While there are sadly many contributing factors to the time we take off – financial, family commitments, etc. – where possible take as much time as you need with the mindset of no deadlines or expectations. We all set our own calendars of grief. Time off to reflect can absolutely either be what our heart requires or leave us feeling lost further – you can make the decision for your own personal requirements. And if any employer is reading this, I beg you to please consider your employee's workload, to be patient with them and gentle on their delicate heart.

Losing a baby is a trauma that extends beyond home. It is carried with us wherever we travel and that includes our work space.

You are faced with the task of finding your new place in the world. Our very identity is altered once we lose a child. I was once the small girl with colourful hair, now I'm the girl whose baby died. We all label others, it's really just a part of our human nature, but you have the power to redesign your label over time, to own it and wear it with pride. You do not just have to be the girl whose baby died, you can be the girl who continued to celebrate her baby long after you lost them, the girl who raised money in memory, the girl who shared her experience with others and helped others to understand. Choose your label and run with it. It doesn't have to be a big public label, it can be whatever you want, it can simply be 'mother' and 'memory keeper'.

Losing our baby rattles us, it jolts us from one imagined future and forces us to realise a new one. It is a future that we want to reject but we will, with time, come to accept. In the meantime we may feel ourselves floundering, or panicked. From the moment that test read positive, we had envisioned ourselves as mothers, and mothers still we are, but our new life is not the one of our dreams. Death of any kind can encourage us to confront the reality of life, its fragility and uncertainty. We find ourselves questioning our beliefs, and wondering how and why this trauma came into our lives. Soul-searching becomes engrained in the bereaved.

While we may never really come to understand the nature of life and death, there is one thing we can be certain of – that life goes on, and it goes on with your baby forever a part of it.

As you step out into the world with your loss heavy in your heart you can:

❋ Expect that there will be times within your day when you will be confronted with your loss – allow yourself to grieve at these times.

❋ Keep your support circle close. There is no need to forever dismiss those who don't understand or 'step up' to comfort, but for now just focus on those who do.

❋ Find some routines and rituals that help you feel close to your baby.

❋ If possible, only return to work when you feel you are ready. Talk to your employer beforehand and lean on friends within your workspace.

❋ Find something that reminds you of your baby, such as a colour, animal or flower, and share this reminder with loved ones, giving them opportunities to embrace your baby's memory alongside you.

EVERLASTING GRIEF

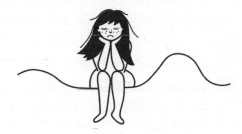

Grief remains one of the most misunderstood emotional journeys of modern times. Even those grieving can struggle to get a handle on it, and those who are yet to truly experience such a deeply personal and all-consuming grief will potentially have real difficulty in grasping it at all. While I do sense a slow shift in the understanding of grief in society, it is still woefully miss-marketed, and grieving the loss of your own baby adds a whole other painful and confusing dimension. It goes without saying that every single person grieves in their own way, there is no right or wrong way to mourn our loss, and while it is simply impossible to write a single chapter tailored for each individual, the basic truths remain universal.

The first thing to get our heads around is the fact that grief is not a passing phase, but rather something we carry with us forever. Sometimes it will feel gritty and dark, a weight that pulls us down into our darkest and loneliest moments, and sometimes it will feel light enough to draw inspiration from. Either way, grief is a journey, an experience, something that remains part of us for our entire lifetime.

If that sounds scary then you can consider that your grief is simply a reflection of your love. Without love there is no grief, and of course you will always love your baby and therefore you will always grieve. Grief lasts forever because love lasts forever. I don't really believe in a 'grieving period', in fact I think we should rub this phrase out the Western dictionary and be done with it. The idea that when someone dies we grieve for a bit, gradually feel better and then eventually heal is painfully misleading, and yet it still often remains the expected norm. Phrases like 'time is a healer' and 'the first year is the worst' are neither truthful nor helpful for a person grieving their baby.

Our grief is fluid. It fluctuates, rises and falls, with passing anniversaries and milestones. Sometimes it exists only as background noise, a soft ongoing hum, other times we are at the mercy of an entire full volume concert.

This doesn't mean you must brace yourself for a lifetime of absolutely agonising grief, but it does mean we can prepare ourselves to let go of the notion that it will end. We are grieving when we sit soaked in tears on the nursery floor, we are grieving when we laugh with our friends. Sometimes an all-consuming pain, sometimes a gentle ache, but always it is there. The notion that grief is a phase, something to push through until we reach the other side, is utterly misplaced. We can begin to accept that grief has no finish line, when we lose our baby there will never be a moment when we are finished grieving, never will the time come when we say 'I'm OK now, I'm not sad about my loss anymore'. You will never 'get over' the loss of your baby, and that is OK.

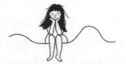

To those around you there is a need to fix things, and grief can be seen as a problem to solve. But, of course, the grieving know that you cannot solve a broken heart just as you cannot replace a missing loved one. There is no solving grief, there is only experiencing grief. It's difficult for those around us to witness, particularly when they are dealing with their own grief too.

Some people may shy away from your grief, too intimidated by the feat of comforting a bereaved parent, too frightened to be reminded of their own mortality, too wary of saying or doing the wrong thing.

We have to make our own personal choices on how we react to those we lose among the shattered remains of our loss, but I'm always aware of the magnitude of such an emotional bombshell and the difficulty some people will ultimately have in navigating that. In other words, there are some friends or family that may never be able to help comfort us because of their own emotional limitations. No one ever expects a baby to die and no one really expects a pregnancy to end in its infancy. No one is ever prepared to deal with it. We can never truly expect others to understand our personal pain, and while there are likely to be some friends and family we can turn to at any moment, there are also likely to be relationships left behind after loss.

When our whole world is altered so drastically, we may discover that some friendships are no longer so easily compatible. My experience of this is that a huge event can pull people apart, but that time and space can bring them back together. It is easier to not write people off altogether, and instead to put them aside with the understanding that the loss of a baby is devastating in many more ways than just the obvious black and white.

We may face hurtful comments. There is the usual role call: 'Everything happens for a reason', 'God needed another angel', 'It wasn't meant to be' and, perhaps the most hurtful, 'At least it happened early on'. When comments like this are thrown around, it is our duty to reply with gentle honesty and a good intention, to explain carefully why these statements aren't comforting. People say these things because they don't know what else to say.

It's not easy — comments like these inflict huge amounts of pain. While we could easily reply with anger, we are likely to lose a friend and they are likely to be left feeling awful. If it is possible, we can take time after the comment to gather our thoughts rather than responding immediately. Comfort was offered but it was not received, we can now take the chance to honour our babies by talking openly and providing the chance for both parties to reflect. You can see this as part of your baby's lasting legacy; to educate, alter perspectives and deepen understanding. Our babies are at it again, teaching those around us about life and death.

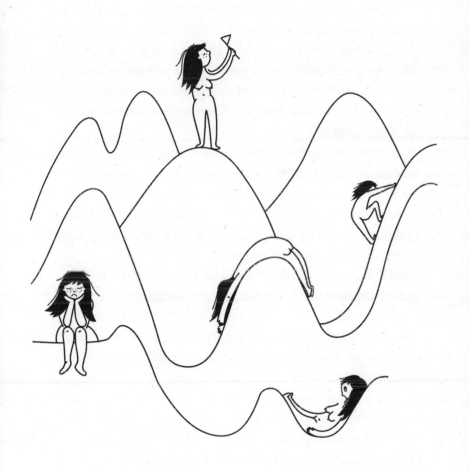

You can build a positive relationship with your grief. There is a saying, 'Grief is just love with no place to go', and it's spot on. In this sense, you can remember that grief is a necessity, your baby is important to you and they deserve your love and that is inclusive of your grief. It is incredibly difficult to manage at times, a searing burn that demands attention, but always, even at its most painful, it exists because of the love you have for your baby. It is part of your connection to your baby.

There is no right way to live with grief, but it is undeniable that we will be living with grief for the rest of our lives now, and so we can begin to accept that we will have 'good moments' and 'bad moments', but neither are right or wrong. I found that people often commented about how strong I was when I was fundraising and writing uplifting and inspirational posts, but at times when I was feeling drowned and missing my son so deeply, I was met with 'chin up' comments or advised to speak with a therapist. Of course, therapy is absolutely a sensible path when grieving, but really it felt as though when I was upset I was considered to be 'weak'.

What I came to realise over time was that grieving in all its aspects takes great strength, and weak and strong are not mutually exclusive. When I was working with charities I was strong, when I cried on the nursery floor clutching my baby's empty clothes I was strong. And so are you. Because it takes strength to accept those painful feelings into your heart and to face the devastating fact that your own flesh and blood has died.

When I miscarried I hibernated, I wanted to be as
physically invisible as I felt. That was not weak, that was
recognition of what my heart required; that wasn't me
escaping, it was me *taking refuge*. Confronting grief with all
its harsh realities is strong, allowing yourself to feel weak is
strong, just living takes strength when you lose your baby.
You may come to realise that you do not want to part with
your grief as it is united with your baby, and we ultimately
hold tight anything that connects us with them.

Your grief is representative of your love. It is natural,
part of your baby's legacy and a piece of them you will
always carry with you.

Something noticeable within the world of the grieving
is the shift in other people's attitude over time. I remember
when my baby boy first died there was an overwhelming
outpouring of love from people close to us. The death of
a newborn baby was just too sad to comprehend, people
sent messages of love, gifts in his memory, his nursery was
decorated in cards and flowers. It was in the immediate
aftermath that people around me felt his loss the greatest.
And yet my own personal experience was one of initial shock
and muddled denial. Motivated by the love for my son and in
a state of disbelief, I felt numb to the pain. In the beginning
my grief was raw yet gentle, I woke up crying and I fell asleep
crying. Those early days of grief were both devastating and
proactive all at the same time, heartbroken yet motivated to
continue his legacy. Of course everyone's experience differs,

but I was so protected by shock that I barely cried at my own baby's funeral, and yet a few weeks into life with our newborn baby daughter I found myself so choked by grief I was literally gasping for air. I needed support in the initial first days, yes, and I also still need it years later.

But I slowly found that people's attitudes to my grief altered over time. What began as 'call me anytime' and 'you're doing so well' slowly hardened into confusion and 'perhaps you should see a doctor'. When friends saw me feeling low and asked what was wrong, I wanted to scream, 'My baby died and he's still dead. Time has passed but I'm still hurting.' I know they meant well, but grief is so ongoing, it is relentless and repetitive. You may begin to feel increasingly left behind.

Just a few weeks after Winter died I distinctly remember seeing my Facebook feed awash with friends' nights out and daft throw-away updates, and I genuinely wondered how the hell everyone else could go about life so nonchalantly. Had they forgotten my baby was dead? How could the world be so insensitive and carry on so brazenly while I was destined to always live a life without my child? Grief does ultimately bring with it an element of selfishness, after all we are the only ones so entirely absorbed in our own world, and life for others does, quite rightly, go on. Regardless, this experience can leave you feeling isolated and angry.

When you grieve you want the whole world to grieve with you, your baby is so important and their loss so monumental.

At times when I was feeling this loneliness, as though no one else cared *enough*, I thought instead about others around me who had lost a loved one. I took a moment to think about how my experience of their loss was different to their own experience in that moment – I had carried on living my life while theirs had forever changed, but still I had thought of them often and reached out at times. When your baby dies, you are the first crack in the ice, you are at the centre of the loss. But that crack extends, it continues to fragment and blister, and continually those around you are affected in one way or another, it is just so difficult to see when our own bubble is so clouded and fogged with our own personal pain. Those around you don't forget, they are simply living a different experience to you. They are not living the same experience and so they cannot feel the same experience and vice-versa. They do not *feel* it the same, so they cannot *live it* the same.

There is a saying 'Grief is the price we pay for love' and of course our babies are so deeply and unconditionally loved that our grief will continue to exist as long as we do. When we really consider it, love always ends with grief. We love those around us knowing that we will one day be separated by death, and yet still we choose to love them. Why? Because the experience of that love is worth the pain in the ending, our grief is the legacy of our love. Here are some tips to help you make sense of your grief:

✱ Remain confident in your knowledge that there is no right or wrong way to grieve.

* Remove time limits and expectations on your grief.
* Take this opportunity to gently educate those around you. When a friend misjudges your emotions and can't understand your pain, you can explain it to them. If someone makes a comment that doesn't sit well with your grief, you can tell them.
* Remember that grief is love, grieving isn't *negative*, it is necessary.

JOY OVER
JEALOUSY

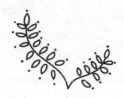

Jealousy is an emotion we have all encountered over the
years, and the loss of our baby can invite this feeling into our
lives by the bucketload. Jealous of pregnancy announcements,
birth announcements, jealous of those around us with
heaving bumps and arms laden with tiny babies, jealous of
how easy it is for everyone else and their smooth and painless
transition into motherhood. It is such an all-consuming
and downright ugly feeling that it inevitably comes hand in
hand with shame, and it is a feeling that we would love to rid
ourselves of entirely, or at least relieve a little where possible.
In this chapter, I'm going to explore where this jealousy comes
from and then look at how to work on eliminating it.

    Firstly, let's not feel shameful of our jealous feelings.
By noting them, you are already taking steps to confront
and change your way of thinking and that is always a
commendable thing. By being proactive, you are honouring
your baby in yet another way. You are embracing their short

life by exploring ways to change your thoughts and feelings for the greater good.

And you are certainly not alone. Jealousy is everywhere in our world, and of course this includes the emotional minefield of the baby loss world, where it is magnified among the emotional blow out of such an intense trauma. Every single human on earth knows jealousy well, whether experiencing the repercussions from someone else who feels jealous or living with the uncomfortable feeling ourselves. 'How many times have you felt jealous?' is an impossible question to answer. Even if as adults we haven't suffered with strong jealousy, there are countless times we experienced it growing up and there are always future opportunities for it to arise, even in the most subtle of ways. And just as we love and grieve with such a deep and strong intensity when our baby dies, we also experience heightened 'negative' emotions such as jealousy. It is part and parcel of the animalistic continuance that our baby's presence brought with it. Their brief life seasoned your own with lashings of emotions, and sometimes they are just harder to navigate than others.

Whether we have lost a baby or not, we know jealousy. When we have lost a baby, we just know it better.

You can begin by realising it not shameful to admit your jealousy, it is in fact rather honourable that you are beginning the journey of relieving yourself of its poisonous burden, all while you keep your baby in your heart.

The first thing I always consider is that jealousy, although a valid and real emotion, is a wasted and pointless sentiment. By feeling jealous of someone else's happiness or success, it doesn't make you feel better and it doesn't stop them feeling happy or being successful. In that sense it is a double loss – you feel worse, they are still happy. Once you realise how empty and worthless the mental pain of jealousy is, you can make a rational and firm commitment to dispose of it.

So why do we feel jealous? Well, simply put, we feel jealous when we feel like our own needs are not met. This feeling comes from our deep-rooted 'self-cherishing', the mentality that all humans possess that puts themselves as their number one priority. We don't need to be ashamed to admit that we have this mindset – we all do, it is our greatest flaw as humans, and it leads to all our subsequent feelings of anger, attachment, jealousy, etc. It is the mindset that subsequently leads humans into division, war and other disastrous situations.

To give an example of this mentality, we can use an analogy: imagine you are walking down your street and you notice that all the houses have smashed windows. Our mind instantly thinks, *Oh wow, I hope MY house hasn't had its windows smashed*. While of course we may feel natural compassion for our friends and neighbours, we are ultimately relieved when we discover that *our* house is OK. Now, imagine that you are told that only one house on your street has been broken into – our self-cherishing leaps in again and says, *I hope it's not*

MY house! Self-cherishing is the mind that values *my* things greater than it values others', whether that be *my* house, *my* car, *my* family, *my* idea, *my* religion or *my* country. It is not to be confused with selfishness, but is rather a naturally arising mindset that promotes strong attachment to 'me, my, mine'.

Jealousy arises from this self-cherishing, it is a feeling that says, *My wish not to suffer is more important than your happiness.* When we read a pregnancy announcement and retreat into jealousy, we are thinking about *our* pain rather than the other person's happiness. In that sense, we are putting our own pain first. We have reverted to our common human flaw that I am more important than you, my feelings are more important than yours. But remember, no self-judgment, no shame. Jealous feelings are entirely natural when your baby dies and other babies live. There is inevitably the feeling that after so much raw pain we have to protect our own heart, and I am not suggesting anyone denies themselves that privilege – I would certainly never suggest you beat yourself up for feeling that way.

Just like you, my life is not devoid of jealousy. I am a human, one who has suffered the loss of her child shortly after he was born and two further losses, and has lived with the subsequent sting of pregnancy and birth announcements. I would like to share with you a personal moment when I felt the rages of jealousy.

I had just suffered my second miscarriage following the sudden death of my newborn son and we were in the run up to his first birthday and anniversary of his death. I was

heartbroken and losing hope when a close friend of mine
announced – quite out of the blue – that she was expecting
a baby. She sent me a beautiful and well-considered text
and I've no doubt she was aware that the news would bring
with it a level of pain for me. But despite knowing all that,
I read the message and my chest burned. I felt angry, I felt
incredibly jealous, and I went straight to bed and cried a river.
My mind said, *Why can she have a baby so easily but I can't?!* In
that moment my pain was more important than the fact that
my friend had just discovered that she was about to become a
mother and was overjoyed at such a life-changing moment. I
instantly thought, *I want that!* rather than, *SHE is deserving of
that happiness.*

Grief is complicated and you must allow yourself to
engage in self-care and be gentle on your heart, but we must
also remember that we are just one single person while others
are countless, and everyone around us deserves happiness.
Yes, we wish with all our hearts that our own baby had this
chance at life, of course we do, but they didn't, their chance at
life has sadly been and gone. In shunning another baby in the
wish for our own to be revived we are simply wishing for the
impossible, and causing ourselves huge pain in the meantime.
It doesn't mean we don't find these situations painful and
want to crawl into a corner and lick our wounds, but it also
means that we can accept that the happiness of others is just
as important as the respect we deserve for our own grief.

I realised eventually that I didn't want my friend – or
anyone – to feel guilty for their happiness. I didn't want her
pregnancy and motherhood to be tainted by my personal

pain. She was happy and why shouldn't she be? I remembered the feeling from my first carefree pregnancy and what a wonderful gift it was for her to experience and rejoice in that. We can all draw from the memories our babies gifted us. Even the briefest of pregnancies harvested a little life so precious and celebrated, our babies taught us what an incredible honour it is to be in that position and so we can recognise the honour of that in someone else too.

You do not need to suppress the feeling of jealousy, you do not need to torture yourself for it. You can simply notice its arrival, challenge why you feel that way, and slowly overcome it.

Another point to contemplate is that we are all on our own journey. If your friend becomes pregnant, has that robbed you of your own chance? Absolutely not. Her – and anyone else's – happiness is not related to yours in that sense. And so, when we really consider this, does it actually make any sense to not feel happy for her? Another healthy baby has an opportunity at life, and that doesn't make or break your own chance at motherhood. The same goes for any situation, our lives are all dependent upon individual circumstances arising, and so we can celebrate the happiness of others as if it were a success of our own.

We can remember that another person feeling happy doesn't mean that we can't be happy. Nobody is capable of stealing your happiness.

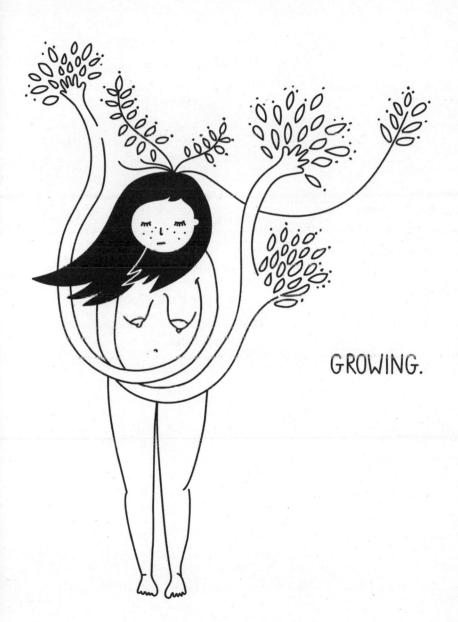

GROWING.

When we are in the throes of loss it can feel as though happiness and suffering have been unevenly distributed, as though there is a limited currency to stretch among us all, and we are left poor. We see others rolling around, rich in happy coins, while we sit alone with our own meagre supply. When we see happiness in this way, we are forgetting that no one is stealing our coins, there is no set amount, there is no limit. It is possible for any of us to be rich this way, regardless of how much the other person next to us has. We may not be feeling such happiness in this present moment, but the future is yet to greet us. To be jealous of those around us who have the happiness we desire in the present moment is denying that future before it even has chance to reach out a hand. Others may have what we want right now, but one day it's possible that we will have what they want.

Often when we feel jealous we discover that this feeling vanishes when we achieve our own happiness, and if this is the case then we can see that jealousy is simply dependent upon our own mind in that moment and therefore it is impermanent. One day here, one day not.

Just because you feel jealous today, doesn't mean you will always feel this way. Our mind shifts and

*changes constantly and we can make the decision as to
which direction we point it, after all it is* our *mind, we
own it.*

There are other countless things to consider. For example, a
stranger who sees me pass by as I hold my baby daughter may
look at me and feel jealous that they do not have a baby. But
of course they don't know my journey to this point. The fact is
that we rarely know a person's full background or history.

A few years ago, I stood in the shop queue, empty womb
and broken heart, behind a heavily pregnant lady, and I
looked at her as if she had the whole world. I thought, *I
want that.* But of course everyone suffers in life, mentally,
physically, emotionally. Was the woman in front of me happy?
Who knows. Perhaps she faced redundancy from her job, no
longer loved her partner or suffered from anxiety. It's easy
to compare suffering and feel as though ours is worse, and
of course I can agree that baby loss is severely cruel, but
suffering is suffering, and no one escapes it for a lifetime, no
one. When I looked at her as if she had the whole world, there
are others looking at me and thinking the same. We only have
to turn on the news and witness the devastation that exists
alongside us in this world to see that we – in our safe-roofed,
cosy and warm, war-free, full-bellied worlds – are objects of
jealousy too.

If we know of others around us in the loss community – or beyond – who are feeling jealous, then we should also know that this requires great compassion from us. Jealousy is so often hurled as an insult, and with it comes a huge amount of personal attack and negative insinuation. But if we all think about a moment when we have felt jealous, then we can easily realise just how ugly it feels. When we are jealous we are angry, ashamed and most likely comparing our personal value to the value of others. It is such a consuming emotion that it is quickly out of our control, and many crimes of passion have been committed by someone who feels jealous.

While it doesn't always mean we are going to turn into a crazed murderer, jealousy can lead us to cut contact with friends and family and say and do tremendously hurtful and regretful things. There is never any good that comes from a feeling of jealousy, and it feels painful and poisonous. No one has ever said 'I love feeling jealous, it's so wonderful!', and those around us who feel jealous are suffering great mental pain. When we do retaliate in jealousy, it feels good for a short time but it is quickly chased by feelings of shame and guilt – if we know how this feels, then we can realise that those around us suffering from jealousy do not require shaming and mocking, but actually they require great compassion to relieve them of such a terrible feeling.

It may take hours, days, weeks, years, to overcome such intense jealousy, but with practice and your baby close in your thoughts, it is possible. And the greatest things happen from those moments where you put it aside – you relieve yourself of the added and wasted suffering of jealousy at a time when you already feel the relentless grip of grief, and you celebrate your friends' happiness. It's not always easy, but as long as you have a mind it is possible.

And so when you feel the green-eyed monster creeping in, remember:

* Jealousy is a natural feeling, no shame in that.
* Jealousy is not a permanent feeling, you will not always feel this way.
* It is a mindset that simply robs you of any happiness for others and therefore you can make a determination to ease or overcome it, with your baby in your heart.
* Somebody else having a baby doesn't steal your own chance of one day holding a living baby of your own.
* Your baby taught you what an incredible honour it is to be pregnant, and how you wish for your baby to be forever celebrated. You can take this lesson they so kindly gifted you and pass it on to a fellow pregnant mother, in your baby's memory.

FACING
NEW LIFE

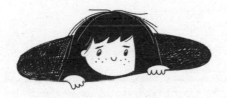

Meeting new babies once you have lost your own is a
challenge, and it is a challenge that comes loaded with fear,
embarrassment, guilt and shame. Something that once
came easy is now a trigger for your own personal grief and
a reminder of all that you have lost. It is a situation that
gives rise to a wealth of complex emotions, an event that
can feel deeply difficult to navigate and almost impossible
to communicate. But you can do it, it's possible, and it's
even possible to enjoy it. With your baby held tightly in your
thoughts, you can make sense of your feelings, take time to
reflect and begin to meet other babies with a gentle heart.

When facing a new baby, the first emotion that springs
to mind is fear. It's a funny one to realise that the prospect of
meeting a tiny harmless baby can be so staggeringly fearful.
And yet it is scary. To the heart of a bereaved mother, facing
new life can leave us awash with fear. So what are we afraid
of? Well get yourself a pen and paper and write the list ... it's
pretty much endless, right?

We are afraid of the unknown, afraid of how we will react, afraid of being judged by others and afraid of our ability to keep it together. We are afraid that our hearts will visibly shatter and our grief will erupt like a heated volcano. And maybe we are afraid that we will be fine and wonder if that is somehow a betrayal to our own baby.

Some encounters with new babies are always going to be more intense than others. A social media friend who is separated by screen, and possibly several hundred miles, could be much easier to congratulate on their new baby than someone we hold close in our hearts. When it is someone within touching distance it feels more real and therefore more intrusive to our grieving.

Some meetings are sprung on us with little warning and we are left thinking on our feet. Those were always the most panic-inducing for me, when I had to rush to gather together my emotions with a pounding heart. In that instant we encounter the famous 'fight or flight' feeling, and the sharp wobbly desperation to escape lickety-split. Overcoming our anxieties takes time, and even in the far future we may find ourselves dropped in the ocean and treading water as we are faced suddenly with a new baby. We will possibly always be flung back to a memory of holding our own, whether that was in our arms or in our womb.

In these situations there is no failure in protecting your heart and making a polite exit. But also you can take some deep breaths to calm your racing mind and maybe, just maybe, you can stay. You can think, *Just two minutes*, and give yourself tiny targets. When two minutes have passed and you are still standing, you can think, *Just two more minutes.* You can leave at any moment, no self-judgment, but you might also surprise yourself and spend a little longer around the baby than you had expected. In these panicky moments I always found it helpful to remember the bravery my son showed in his brief life and follow his lead – he fought so hard to stay with us. Our babies demonstrated great courage by simply striving to exist.

Even the briefest of flourishes is a show of great strength, a reminder of how daring our babies were. They taught us to embrace life in all its scary challenges. We can learn from the example they so brazenly set.

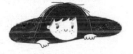

The next feeling that we may experience is an uncomfortable sense of embarrassment. It sits well alongside our misplaced shame. Mixed in with the blazing pressure to *keep it cool*, our embarrassment can stem from an underlying feeling of failure. Here you are, presented by someone who has *successfully* brought a baby into the world. There is a feeling of being left behind. An experience that you had shared up until a certain point has come to an end and you are now venturing out into different territories, your own carefree journey cruelly cut short. Now here you stand with cemented feet while your friend runs on ahead, so far removed from your own stumbling point they have become lost on the horizon, a blur of triumph for us to squint at. We have been overtaken, someone else is living the life we had set out to achieve. A sense that they have *won* where we have *lost*.

Meeting their baby, particularly alongside other family and friends, feels like we are the losers in a competitive sport about to be paraded in front of the winning team. Embarrassment that we are *not good enough*, and while they stand there polishing their well-deserved trophy, we are left starkly empty handed. But our embarrassment, although a valid feeling, is heavily unfounded. Losing a baby is out of our hands, it is something we have no control over, we have not failed. The very fact that you have scooped yourself up and chose to celebrate your baby in whatever way you feel possible, is honourable, brave and worthy of some serious self-congratulation.

You don't need to feel embarrassed, you can instead feel proud. Your life has taken a monumental change of direction, and yet here you are, positively working through the scattered emotions and taking sturdy steps to meet your friend's baby.

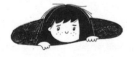

There is the rise of grief that comes with meeting a new life. That deep burning desire to hold *your* baby. It is inevitable, as you are faced head on with all the pain that came with your own baby's death. It is unfortunate that meeting other new babies can be a trigger in your own personal suffering, and in those moments it is incredibly difficult to see past anything other than your blistering hurt. Even if you navigate the meeting with reasonable success, in the aftermath you can find yourself flung back into the early days of raw grief.

It's as though you are walking a dangerous path, treading lightly, avoiding the potholes and dragging yourself up the hills, and facing new babies is a tumble down a muddy trench. You have to find the energy to somehow pull yourself out once more, but first, maybe it's OK if you take some time to sit in the dirt. You might feel like you are going backwards, but you are not. You are simply learning how to master new experiences following a heartbreaking trauma, and anything that needs to be mastered requires practice. If a meeting doesn't go too smoothly, or if it is sprung on you and you shrink and escape, it's OK. Give yourself a break, chalk it up to experience, know that in these situations you are putting your heart on the line and that is not easy for anyone to do. Life after baby loss presents us with an endless list of difficult events and circumstances and we are thrown into it with no training.

You are human, you have suffered immensely, you are stepping into the unknown with no proven manual and you are trying.

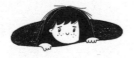

And there are the feelings of guilt. A friend, a loved one, has invited you to meet and hold their baby, and our first gut feeling is, *I don't want to*. It's easy to feel like an awful person. This new life, so innocent, so precious and loved, it's such a special and honourable invite, and here we are, not wanting to go, not wanting to see and touch someone else's baby.

We feel guilty for our initial gut reaction, but we mustn't feel guilty for what are natural and valid emotions. The very fact that they have been thought through, written and compiled into a book by a mother who has lost one baby post birth and two in the very beginnings of pregnancy can assure you of that. And the very fact that these feelings have been universally shared by loss mothers in the wider community can serve as a 'me too'. You can relax with the knowledge that these are thoroughly *normal* feelings experienced by many in similar situations.

Almost everyone I have spoken with in the baby loss community has found meeting new babies to be a challenging situation – even those who have a naturally light attitude have still found times when they have struggled. They are such universal feelings following loss, and you certainly don't need to feel guilty about emotions that are anticipated and expected. Any time a new baby is born it is a highly charged event, such is the nature of this significant human accomplishment. And when you have lost your own baby, you are simply piling a whole load of extra deeply felt emotions on top.

We are talking about raw emotion here, deeply engrained animalistic emotion. Seeing a birth announcement can be enough for us to retreat from social media and send us into a virtual hibernation. Physically meeting a baby can be enough to send your heart crashing to the floor. It hurts; it doesn't just hurt you, it hurts many loss mothers. And of course we feel shameful for our aversion, because no one wants to admit to having negative feelings towards an innocent baby. I know I felt deeply ashamed. How could I feel so ugly towards something so beautiful? But the truth is less frightening. You are not experiencing these emotions because you are to meet a healthy living baby, you experience them because you do not have your own, and these feelings simply arise in the moments you are confronted with that painful reality.

You should never feel ashamed of how you feel, you are not a bad person, you are not a bad friend.

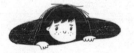

When meeting new babies our mind inevitably plays a huge part. I always found that the events leading up to the meeting were decisive as to how it would go. Has it been a light morning, a peaceful few days, is grief being particularly gentle on your heart? Perhaps we are going through a time when we are overwhelmed with gratitude for our baby's brief life and life is being kind to us. The obstacle of meeting another new baby always feels achievable when our mind and grief are both more relaxed and in tune. But on those darker days where our grief pulls us towards pain, where we feel especially vulnerable and the aching for our baby is greater than any inspirational mindset, those meetings are not always possible. Yes, I have politely declined invites on these days, and so can you.

To begin with, the best option is always to open the conversation with your friend or family member. You know how it feels to live among the deep and complex ruins of life after baby loss, but those around you may or may not have such a clear idea. There may be times when you are purposely left out on invites to meet a friend's new baby, as well as times when you receive an invite that seems completely ignorant to the pain it may inflict on us. You can realise that those around you are often at a loss at what to do, uncertain of how to avoid causing you suffering or feeling awkward and uncomfortable for our foreign situation.

Baby showers and newborn meetings can become a lottery. If we are skipped from the invites we feel shunned and contagious of death, if we are invited we can feel instant anxiety and dread. No one wants to be known at such events as 'the one who's baby died' and yet it is, in some ways, inevitable. The label can make us feel uneasy, as though everyone is watching us very closely for reactions. It's a lot of pressure to suddenly *be* a certain way. And that pressure is ramped up if you haven't spoken about how you will be feeling. Whether your baby died after birth and you had the chance to hold them, or you lost your baby before an announcement and feel as though you harvested a secret that you never had the chance to share, being met with a bump or a baby serves only as a reminder of what you had snatched from you before you could even contemplate a pink or blue cake or a babygrow filled with baby.

I always found the newborn meetings easiest when I could openly talk about how I was feeling, always staying mindful of the other family's immense joy and pride in that moment. If you can just find your voice and send a simple message in advance, the pressure can ease, at least a little. For instance:

> I look forward to meeting your beautiful baby. I just need you to know that holding your baby will be emotional for me, having lost my own. Please don't mistake this for me not joining in your celebration, meeting new babies always reminds me of my own baby. Your baby is so very precious and I thank you very much for the invite. I will see you on Saturday x.

It is possible to be honest and real about how you feel without tarnishing the other person's happiness.

Once again it's important to remember that while you are responsible for your own intentions and actions, you are never responsible for how others react. A good friend will anticipate that this meeting will be a challenge on some level. They will see that once you have held your baby that did not survive, or were even denied that chance, holding their living baby will bring with it some level of pain by association. But other people will, unfortunately, never really 'get it'. That is out of your hands. Maybe with time their understanding will evolve, maybe not. If you have played your part in gently educating and bravely sharing your emotions then you must be proud of yourself and accept it for what it is.

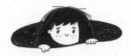

Once you have voiced your nerves and lifted some external pressure, you can work on your own inner pressure too. Much of the worry around meeting other babies comes with our runaway imagination. We often think that our imagination is something left just for children, for them to use in dress up and role play. But as adults we use our imagination day in, day out. We imagine what we will pick up from the supermarket, we imagine what we will wear to an event, we imagine how our weekend will pan out. The human imagination is responsible for every single man-made object and event around us. The house we are living in began in the imagination of an architect, our bedsheets. At dinner time, the plate for our dinner and the recipe for the very meal itself, all began in someone's imagination. Once we start exploring this, we can see just how frequently we use our imagination and just how powerful it is, even for grown-ups.

The problem with imagination, however, is that it doesn't always work in our favour, and at times we need to put effort into harnessing it for the greater good. How many times have we imagined an interview or important meeting going wrong? How many times have we sat up at night worrying, playing over in our head anything and everything that can go wrong? We fool ourselves into believing this ritual is an integral part of our preparation – if we think of all the bad things that could happen then we are somehow ready for them. But actually we are just selling ourselves a story where disaster strikes, and over time we begin to believe that story is the truth. How many times have those past situations actually worked out OK? How many times have we sat down afterwards and thought, *All that worrying for nothing?*

The same goes for when we are preparing to meet another baby. Yes, it may not go completely to plan, you may still be flooded with nerves and you may lose your head a little, but, like so many other experiences we can draw from, we will find that the imagining is often much worse than the actual doing.

Take some time before any baby meetings to imagine it going well.

Find a quiet space, close your eyes, breathe, and imagine that you will face that tiny new baby with some inner confidence. Play the story out positively. Believe it, take it in your stride, it is possible and it may even be enjoyable.

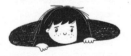

Something interesting to consider is the experience from the other person's perspective. Do you remember how excited you were in your own pregnancy and the subsequent pride you have for your own baby? Your friend is feeling this too.

I faced some difficulty when announcing the pregnancy that evolved into my daughter. Knowing it was a delicate topic in the world of loss and trying to conceive, I privately messaged those I was close to within the loss community 'pre-warning' of my announcement. As expected, I received a mixed bag of replies – while some were thrilled for me, there were equally many who were so consumed by their own suffering that they could not celebrate my news. No judgment here, I know how deep that pain runs, which is exactly why I chose to announce privately first. But there was a conflict within myself and in hindsight I can see I didn't always react as gracefully as I had hoped, and this experience gave me another fresh perspective.

When I was left feeling guilty for my happiness, as though I wasn't allowed to celebrate and undeserving of my good news despite all the pain I had suffered in my journey beforehand, I realised this is how I could have ended up making others feel when they had previously announced a pregnancy to me. Those around us who give birth to a healthy live baby could be left feeling these same emotions.

Not every baby is a baby born after loss, but all babies are special regardless. If it is too difficult for you to join in their celebration then that is OK, but alongside this you can remember that they are entitled to celebrate.

NOT YET READY TO COME OUT.

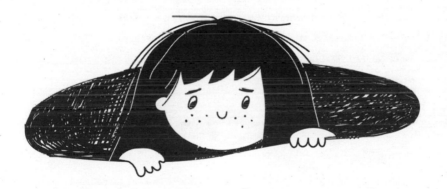

Perhaps it's too hard on your heart to muster the strength to meet the baby, and that is OK. You could always balance it out with a heartfelt text, a simple:

> Congratulations on the birth of your gorgeous baby
> and thank you for the invite to meet her. I'm sorry
> to say that my heart still feels very heavy with
> my own loss, and I'm not able to join you just yet.
> Nevertheless I'm thrilled she has arrived safely and I
> wish you and your family all the best. x

If you can remember how warm it feels when someone close to you tells you how beautiful your baby was – and still is – then we can recognise that this feeling goes for parents of living babies too.

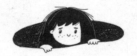

Once it comes to the physical act of meeting and holding a baby, your reaction may surprise you. Will you think of your own baby in that moment? Of course. While you may find a way of separating some parts of the encounter from any memories of your own, you will naturally be recalling any personal experiences or the longing for your arms to be filled; you would be inhuman not to. But in meeting a new baby, you are not betraying the baby you lost, nor are you damaging your own chances at filling your arms one day in the future. While any of these darker emotions and inner conflicts are valid, you can recognise that they simply serve to heap pain and suffering on top of your already broken heart. Instead you can begin to see that this new baby symbolises life, and just as you wish to celebrate the life of your own baby – however brief – you can celebrate the life of another. In fact I'm sure your own baby would be gently willing you on with pride, reminding you just how important it is to have your baby's existence recognised and celebrated; you can give this gift to your friend.

So when stepping out to face new life, remember:

✻ It's OK to feel afraid, you can draw strength from the courage of your baby.
✻ You don't need to feel ashamed or embarrassed, your feelings are natural and valid.
✻ If you can voice how you feel it can relieve some pressure.
✻ Facing new life is a challenge, it is all part and parcel of your new life, and with time and practice you can master it.
✻ If it's too much of a leap to begin with, you can opt out of the meeting and still allow the other person to celebrate.
✻ Your imagination can fool you into expecting the worst. Take some time to believe in the best.

EASING
THE ANGER

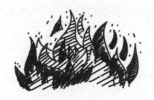

Anger is a natural part of our grief journey, it is a valid and understandable emotion to experience when you are left feeling so cheated and empty. But harvesting huge amounts of anger can also cause unnecessary pain and draw much negativity around your lost baby's memory, and so it can be useful to let go of some anger and practice ways of managing what remains.

To begin with, we can look at the roots of anger, the damage it can cause and its fundamentally futile quality. As someone with a keen interest in Buddhism, I discovered rich solace in a teaching on the subject of anger that I would like to share with you. Buddha taught that holding on to anger is like drinking poison and expecting the other person to die. In other words, feeling angry has no real benefit, offers no solution and simply serves to harm ourselves and bring along with it suffering and pain. Much like taking a clean glass of water and filling it with mud, when we feel angry we are polluting our mind with a thick fog in which our whole world becomes unclear; it robs us of clarity.

Anger is such a heated emotion, it erupts in our belly, it pounds our heart, it chokes us. When we feel so consumed by this anger it's almost impossible to make a clear and informed decision.

Imagine if something, anything, upsets you and you sit and feel angry about it. Does the anger alter the situation? By feeling angry have you resolved the problem? While your anger may motivate you at times to take action, and there may be circumstances where action needs to be taken, there is not enough motivation in the world that can revive and return your lost baby. No amount of anger will deliver them back into your arms. And therefore you can see that anger is only harmful and not at all proactive. That feeling of deep frustration arises because things simply aren't the way we want them to be, and no matter how much we invest in this mindset, things will *never* be how we want them to be. We are simply left in the same situation and feeling angry.

No one floats through baby loss with only gratitude and inspiration, it's not possible, but anger is one feeling we can all look to reduce. Such an ugly, churning emotion, it is true that keeping hold of anger quickly transforms into a form of reckless self-punishment – something that so many of us loss mothers are unfortunately particularly good at.

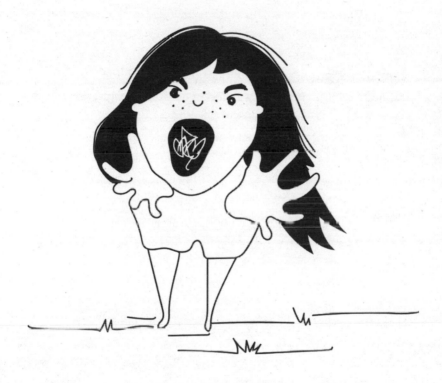

I AM ANGRY.

So, why do we feel angry when we have lost our baby? What triggers our anger? What is it directed at and how can we work towards overcoming this blazing emotion? Well, first of all this is a list that everyone's own experience dictates, and it is a flexible list at that, forever changing as our grief evolves and shifts and we find new angles to view our situation from. Just as no two grief journeys are the same, there are also no rights and wrongs in the patterns and fluctuations of our other emotions. In this book, I simply explore feelings commonly shared within the loss community.

We feel angry because we feel cheated out of our happy ending.

I have felt this anger so deeply. I birthed my son and had merely dipped my toe into the pond of motherhood when he was torn from me. Nine months of heartburn, aching hips, a stretched back and people saying 'It will all be worth it in the end', only to be left with a broken heart and an empty nursery. My prize had been dangled like a carrot for my entire pregnancy, only to discover that it was, in fact, a mirage. It felt like the biggest case of second prize ever. And the same goes for my miscarriages – excitement and happiness replaced so swiftly by desolate heartbreak.

As loss mothers we feel angry for everything that has been snatched from us. 'Cheated' is absolutely an appropriate description for our feelings. We are angry because it is not how it was meant to be and relief from this anger comes only with some gentle acceptance. Even writing this I'm holding my breath, because I know all too well that acceptance of these painful circumstances feels so impossible at times. Do we ever fully accept that our babies are gone? No, not really. There are days when I question not only if my son's death happened, but even if his life ever happened too. It is so natural to feel angry about this, about our life not being how we want it to be, about our baby's life being cut so cruelly short.

Maybe it is not always possible to sit with a rational mind and search for acceptance, maybe your grief will not always allow it, and that's OK. But in those moments when you need this anger lifting from your shoulders, inviting a little acceptance can offer us some breathing space. If acceptance of your loss is too far away, then maybe just an acceptance of your grief instead. You can find a quiet place, close your eyes, focus on your breath and take a moment to relax yourself a little. Think about your baby and connect with them. You can take time to sit in the *here and now*, holding your baby close in your heart and recognising that you keep them there with such ferocity that their presence is palpable.

Your baby existed, they were real, they continue to be real, their existence is not erased by death, it is simply altered.

We can relieve ourselves of the anger and frustration that comes with continually wishing things were different and the futile nature of pouring our heart into impossibilities. Instead of punishing yourself with what you *can't do* you can instead invite focus on the present moment and regain control of what you *can do*. And you can make a dedication, to take that time and energy wasted on anger, and to instead transform it into something positive as part of your baby's lasting legacy.

You may feel angry that your body failed you. As a woman it seems our most natural job is to grow and birth a baby. There is such a distinct feeling of incompetence, of personal failure, like our body did not meet its most basic and expected standards in growing a healthy baby. And those misplaced thoughts of, *What did my body do wrong?* inevitability translates as, *What did I do wrong?* In our confusion we become frustrated and angry, so angry that we somehow disappointed ourselves, let ourselves down and were responsible in some way for the death of our dependent baby. We need to find a way to quieten these false voices of failure.

So, firstly there is no failure in growing a baby that could not stay. Was your baby not perfect in every way even after death? However little or long we carried them for, they are simply always a perfect creation.

When you feel as though you failed, you can remember that your body provided you with an entirely immaculate being, a spectacular and unblemished baby. Whether they were able to stay with you or not, there was nothing wrong with them, they were perfectly right.

Looking around, you can quickly appreciate the enormity of the loss community. So many babies, so many mothers, so many dads, so many families. Such a vast amount of medical

reasons for loss and simply a huge amount of pregnancies
that never transformed into living breathing babies. Are all
these women failures? Did all these babies fail? Fail is such
an awful and self-accusatory word. How can we say we have
failed when we loved our babies so deeply? There is no such
thing as a fail because there is no such thing as a failed loving
mother. If you were to meet another fellow loss mother who
said, 'It's my fault my baby died,' you wouldn't hesitate to
assure them, from a place of truth, that it is undeniably not
the case. In fact it would seem almost ridiculous for her to
be so full of self-blame. Being a good friend to her, you would
take the time in leading her to realise that nothing took her
baby's life except the course of life itself. Give yourself a break
— be that good friend to yourself.

As well as this, we can rationalise that building a whole
new human from scratch is far from simple. Creating an
entire person is a task so powerful and fragile that it remains
mostly beyond our human comprehension. Our wombs house
tiny miracles with every single spark of life. And wherever
there is life there is chance of death. That is a fact that we
so easily forget, and one that our babies reminded us of – the
preciousness, the fragility, the indefinite *gift* of life. Growing
a baby is, sadly, one of life's ultimate natural lotteries, never
promised and never guaranteed.

We are learning slowly, as baby loss and fertility taboos
are broken and conversation around such topics opens
up, that being pregnant, growing and birthing a baby
are all absolutely mammoth tasks in terms of natural
accomplishment. Modern science and medicine is involved

in the creation and growth of millions of babies all around the world every single day. Growing and birthing a baby is natural, yes, but it often requires intervention and a helping hand. Not all rests upon our bodies and it is not ever as easy as just falling pregnant, kicking back and simply trusting in a fruitful outcome. When we consider the feat of conjuring up an actual little life and placing them on earth (no matter how brief a visit) our human heads just cannot comprehend all the magical mechanics behind it.

Every baby is an epic creation so complex and unique that it outwits and fascinates even the greatest philosophers and scientists the world over. You cannot ever hold yourself and your body entirely responsible for such an intricate and untamed masterpiece.

You may feel the rise of anger when you see others around you with living babies complaining, or seemingly taking their children for granted. You may feel a sense of injustice, that you would love a baby so intensely and yet they are so flippant and ignorant to the great prize they possess. While stories in the news of child neglect may have always been particularly painful to hear, now we also find it difficult to read a friend's Facebook post protesting at their lack of sleep with a newborn. In these and similar circumstances the urge to react in anger and resentment is fierce. To shout, 'Don't complain, that's what I WANT!'

It is never easy to see others being dismissive of something that we feel we see a greater value in. We might feel as though others are in possession of a precious treasure without realising its worth, but the likelihood is they do. As loss mothers we just feel *so incredibly deeply* at times. In these moments, remember that your experiences in life have shaped your views and opinions, your loss has lead you to have an intensified outlook. Those throwaway statuses and comments are not aimed at you directly. They are written by a mother, just like you, overwhelmed by the responsibilities and commitments that come with their version of motherhood. They may be complaining about challenges you wish to face, but that doesn't make those challenges invalid, you simply have an alternative and heightened perspective. A mother complaining of waking through the night is a mother who is exhausted. A mother complaining of her toddler's tantrums is a mother struggling to understand the emotional needs of her child.

Motherhood is difficult – dead babies, living babies, mothering in all its diverse glory offers challenges.

Everyone's loss is personal, and I am reminded while writing this that not everyone has a pleasant experience of hospital care, or perhaps you have lost your baby in circumstances of negligence. Wherever there is a possibility of blame there is, of course, likely to be increased feelings of anger and a burning resentment that comes with such a tragic circumstance. Where we have been let down, where the outcome really *could* have been so different, we are inevitably likely to feel anger. In these instances, we may not only harbour anger towards those we feel let us down, but also inaccurately at ourselves. We even feel angry at our past self for not taking action before the tragedy occurred, as though we were somehow irresponsible. We question: *Why didn't I research more, investigate, understand how it could happen, so I could prevent it? Why had we not educated ourselves so we could stop the disaster in its tracks?* We can feel angry at our list of regrets and the resentful gift of hindsight.

You are absolutely allowed to grieve and take time to come to terms with such a painful injustice. Your anger will flare; the very idea that your baby was not fairly offered the chance at life that was available to them is gravely distressing.

To ease some of this anger into proactive healing, honour your baby's life in the most spectacular way possible. Hold their brief life and your loss in your hands and pass it on to other families, making powerful steps to improve available healthcare and deepen the understandings of loss. You can take the failings and the new-found knowledge to voice concerns, raise awareness, campaign where necessary, spread the message and help change to arrive where it is desperately needed. In the moments where you find yourself out of energy and motivation, even the smallest of actions can have a beneficial impact. Even if that is simply sharing an article online to inform others of the signs of a potentially fatal medical condition, or signing a petition for a change in the law for a particular aftercare, such as bereavement therapy as standard or additional support through subsequent pregnancies.

Take that anger and transform it into a loving motivation to save other families from a similar fate. And each night before you climb into bed, you can say, Look what you are doing baby, you are moving mountains, you are a lifesaver.

We cannot save our lost babies, but their lives were not without great meaning. You can use your own loss for someone else's gain, dedicating the benefits to your baby. In this way you are quite literally giving the gift of life to other babies. *Your baby* is giving the gift of life. That is so very special.

Something really beneficial to consider when we feel particularly angry is how we want to immortalise and remember our babies. When I sense anger creeping up on me, I take a photograph of my son and hold it with me in a quiet space. What emotions do I want to carry around with me in my son's memory? What emotions do I want connected to his life? As I study his image, I hold him in my heart. He is so small, delicate, fragile, innocent. The feelings I have for him are nothing but love, endless, boundless love. As mothers, none of us want our baby's memory to include and promote anger. They are too little and pure for that. Instead we want their life and memory to promote the love and meaning they deserve, and so this is the alternative path we can choose to stride down together.

And so, when you want to keep anger at bay, you can:

❋ Take time to be in the here and now. You do not have control over your baby's death, but you do have control over your baby's lasting presence in this world.

❋ Remember your baby was, and forever is, perfect. Your body created that perfect life. Death is out of your hands, but your body gifted you a beautiful and precious baby regardless of how brief their life.

❋ Recognise that motherhood is difficult in all its variations – we are all on our own journeys, we all have our own challenges.

❋ Transform any failings in your care into a loving motivation to raise awareness, create positive change and spread life-saving messages, and dedicate that action to your baby.

❋ Think about what emotions you want connected to your baby's memory, and dismiss those you don't want.

WHY *NOT* ME?

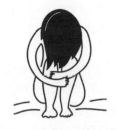

Why ME? It is the question we inevitably ask when faced with difficult circumstances. In those moments of relentless pain we sit inside our own isolated bubble, seemingly surrounded by happy families with living babies. And of course the intense heartbreak of losing a baby inevitably draws us to ask, *Why did this happen to ME?* It is only natural and self-protective, and sometimes, in my personal experience, a little self-indulgence can be exactly what the heart requires in that moment. But for those moments when the *Why me?* weighs heavily on our shoulders, and we feel lonely and detached from the outer world, we can sit instead with the thought, *Why NOT me?*

We don't have to go far to find others who are in pain, and no one escapes suffering for a whole lifetime. It is a tragic inevitably of our very existence.

While there is nothing to gain from competitive grief or deciding who scores higher or lower in the tragedy stakes, it's clear to see that we live surrounded by people suffering at all different levels. We can see suffering in our own living room without even moving from the sofa – just turn on a news channel. Homelessness, depression, bankruptcy, loneliness. Take a walk through a hospital ward. Cancer, dementia, terminally ill children, lives cut short by accident and disaster. Even in the animal realm, forgotten pets left to starve, unwanted pets beaten, others forced to perform; in the wild too, orphaned animals left to fend for themselves, animals caught in nets and traps, or injured from fighting. Pain and suffering is all around us, such is the nature of life.

Undoubtedly, baby loss is a particularly difficult burden to bear and our suffering is not reduced or solved through contemplation alone, but instead we can try to find opportunities for celebration among the devastation, no matter how small. For example, I hold on to the knowledge that I carried my son lovingly in my womb and held him gently in my arms as he died, and that he knew only love in this big tough world. I was there for every big transition, womb to arms and life to death. He died peacefully surrounded by those who care so deeply for him. These are precious moments not experienced by mothers who lose their children in war zones or to a murderous predator.

Instead of torturing myself with the knowledge that my son's brief life was consumed by suffering, the fits and pain he undoubtedly endured in his day long fight for survival, I instead indulge myself in the great fortune of seeing his eyes, something denied to many mothers. And respectfully, I offer to parents who have lost their babies before this opportunity, the reassurance that their child fell asleep peacefully to the lullaby of their mother's heartbeat, having lived a life free from pain and untainted by any ugliness in this world.

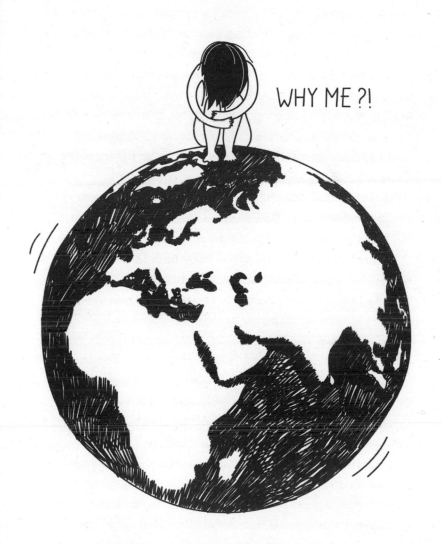

It isn't about who has it easier or harder, or an instruction to 'get on with it' because other people may have it worse. Our grief is huge, important and absolutely valid. But alongside our personal pain we can simply recognise that every single person suffers, and yet here we are, in our millions, and all asking that same question, *Why ME?*

I would like to share with you a popular Buddhist tale that explores the healing qualities of realising the suffering of others:

Many years ago, in an Indian village, lived a woman named Kisa. She was content in her life, happily married and with a newborn baby boy. Then one day her husband became unwell and died. In the throes of grief, Kisa held tightly to her son, but then one day soon after, her little boy also became sick and died.

In denial and unable to accept that her newborn baby had also passed away, Kisa instead imagined he was simply asleep and carried him with her in search of a medicine to cure him. Nobody was able to help her; everyone could see the baby had died, but no one could tell her. Eventually she was told to go and see Buddha himself.

As soon as she met with Buddha he was able to see her tiny bundle had already died, but could see that Kisa was not able to accept it. So instead he offered a suggestion, and sent Kisa to collect mustard seeds to make medicine, with the instruction that

they were only able to come from a home where death
had not taken a loved one.

Kisa dashed off in hope. She visited many houses
that day, and every single house had seeds to offer,
but each time she was not able to take them as the
families shared stories of loved ones they had lost.
A young woman remembered her grandmother who
had recently died, an old man spoke of his daughter
who had died the year before, and a young boy talked
of his father who had died when he was himself just
a baby.

Kisa quickly came to realise that everyone she
met had lost people that they love, everyone had
suffered in grief. In time she recognised that her
baby boy had died, and she found a beautiful garden
in which to lay him to rest, with the new-found
understanding that death is a part of life that touches
us all.

Of course, the death of a baby is different in so many ways to
the death of a grandparent or even a parent. Cheated out of a
full and rich life and denied long-lasting memories, the death
of a baby is out of the natural order and particularly painful
to live through. There is absolutely no denying that. We are
entitled to feel angry and resentful; we have lost something
we never had the chance to fully embrace. But alongside this,
we can also contemplate that death is a part of life that we
have no control over, and it sadly steals loved ones without
a second thought for those left behind. Every single human

on earth is touched by death and the loss of a loved one. In this sense our babies taught us another special lesson, that nothing in life is promised, that we never truly know when we will lose those we love, and we must therefore embrace our family and friends – and strangers too – with open arms.

To contemplate all this suffering around us isn't intended to be depressing, instead it reminds us of the fragility of life and therefore invites greater meaning into our day, reminding us of what we have *rather than what we* have not.

When we see someone suffering with arthritis we discover a new-found appreciation for our flexibility. When we see someone mourning the loss of a parent we feel compelled to hold our own close. When we see someone homeless and cold on the streets we are reminded of how fortunate we are to have a warm house and a comfortable bed to sleep in.

And we can learn from our own heartbreak how to care for others. Experiencing something as traumatic as the loss of a baby throws up an opportunity to nurture our own inner compassion. This is another gift from your baby, the ability to love with an even bigger heart. When we have lost so deeply, we learn to care more deeply too. As you shop, walk, drink in a café, you will be surrounded by silent suffering. We wear our own loss like a silent fog – the strangers we pass have no idea of our magnitude of loss, just as we have no idea of theirs. We can take our own painful experience and

transform it into ways of helping those around us who suffer
too. We suddenly know just how difficult life can be when we
are robbed of the normality that once existed in our happy
bubble. Now instead of passing by a homeless person, too busy
and preoccupied to truly grasp their pain, we will instead
see them as somebody's son or daughter and empathise with
difficulties they encounter in the face of personal tragedy,
regardless of whether that is the familiar loss of a loved one
or the choking grip of addiction.

As with any suffering, we feel our own the greatest. If we
sit at a table surrounded by strangers, all sharing our tales
of pain, our own voice is inevitably always the loudest. While
we may sit and listen and feel deep compassion for another
person's hurt and difficulties, and we may even, with supreme
kindness, offer them help and solutions to help remedy
their suffering, there comes a point where we can stand up
and walk away. We leave them with their problems and we
continue to carry our own, and vice-versa. The suffering
we experience personally always stays with us, we cannot
simply walk away from it, hence why our own feels bigger and
heavier.

When a stranger shares their personal worry with us,
we are never as worried about it as they are. When someone
confides in us that they are worried about an upcoming life
event, maybe an interview or performance, it is so easy for us
to simply say, 'Don't worry you'll be fine!', whereas when we
are the one who is worried, the fear is very real and especially
huge. Our worry, fear, suffering, etc., is often very introverted
in that sense. We own our pain and we carry it with us in our

own little world. Just as it is not possible to put our pain and grief to one side, it is difficult for us to recognise the enormity of suffering in those around us. And yet everyone is suffering, every single person, in one way or another. We can recognise that while we may carry the weight of *Why me?* – we are simply one person surrounded by countless others, all living through life's exceptional highs and ravaging lows. All human. All equal. And all suffering. It is not so much a case of *Why me?*, but instead a case of, *Why us? Why NOT me?*

The ability to recognise suffering, not just within ourselves, but all around us, and to act with compassion to help soothe that suffering, is just another lasting legacy of our babies.

When lost in the loneliness of *why me* try to:

❋ Recall any positive experiences you had with your baby and hold them close, whether the joy at the positive test, the lessons their brief life taught you or holding them in your arms.

❋ Recognise how fortunate you are to be warm, fed, healthy, loved. No, this does not dismiss your grief, you are still allowed to hurt. It simply invites some gentle gratitude and a little light in the darkness.

❋ Contemplate the suffering of all your fellow humans and realise we are *all* suffering in one way or another.

❋ Take another lesson your baby's life taught you with the recognition of others' suffering – the increased capacity for compassion your baby gifted you with.

A MOTHER STILL

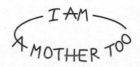

With our arms empty we could be fooled into thinking that we are not included in Mother's Day. But Mother's Day is reserved not just for those with children we can see, but also for those with children we can't. Let's think of it instead as a celebration of motherhood, in all its wobbly variations.

Our first feelings can be of, *Where do I fit in? Do I count as a mother? How can I celebrate the day without my baby here?*

If we have held life in our womb, no matter how briefly, we have at some point been a mother. And once you are a mother, you are always a mother.

To those around us it may seem confusing as to where we draw the line, but it's actually pretty black and white. Are you a mother if you didn't give birth? Are you a mother if your child died without ever taking a breath? Well, yes, of course. Mothers are wise enough to realise that life begins long before birth. We may see the beginnings of our baby on a screen, we may feel their kicks and rolls, we may see our belly swell as it works to house our intended future. In all scenarios we have harvested a life inside us. While we may not feel like a mother in the traditional sense, we are a mother the very first moment we carry that spark of life.

Motherhood is not always about changing nappies and night feeds — these are only a small aspect of what being a mother means. If we look at the bigger picture we can see that being a mother is much more than the physical acts, motherhood is about nurture, and utilising and spreading the love that comes with the title. Just as there are sadly many mothers in the world who are, for some reason or another, unfit in the care of their babies, there are many mothers in the world who are fit for the job but remain empty armed.

If we were to birth and raise a child providing only the bare minimum of food and nappy changes, we would still be called a mother, and yet this is simply not enough to provide a child with all their needs. SO MUCH MORE is required ... care, patience, courage, strength, passion, endless love. The absence of our child cannot remove those qualities from our heart; we still possess the core ingredients of motherhood.

There are so many mothers without children. Whether they have birthed and buried them or are still waiting for that double line, we are still mothers in an unconventional way. It is possible to have the qualification without the experience. In this world of baby loss, a world where we are all striving to achieve this ultimate title, let's first allow ourselves the honour of calling ourselves 'a mother'.

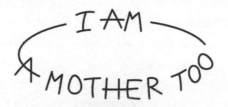

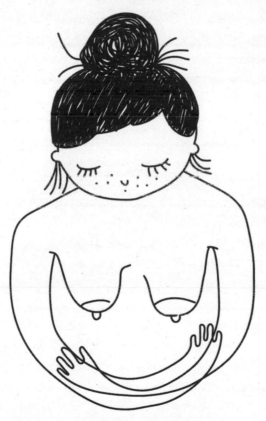

So now, we can hold that title firm. And you know what, we can hold on to it with pride too, because motherhood and pride go hand-in-hand. Have you ever met a mother who is not proud in some way of their child? And we are certainly still proud of ours whether they are visible to the outside world or not. If they battled to stay alive then we are proud of their strength, grit and courage. If they stayed silently in our womb, we are proud of their determination, beauty and the love they gave us. If their life inside us began and ended as swiftly as the sun rises and sets, then we are still proud of the hope they filled our hearts with and the dreams they filled our heads with, and of their gentle and meaningful existence.

We always imagine that as a mother we will spend our lives teaching our children, but they often end up teaching us more, and this is true even of babies that couldn't stay with us. We can take great pride in the fact that our babies gifted us with such meaningful lessons, such as the preciousness of life, the importance of loving those around us and the knowledge that love lives on forever. If we put aside the commercial drive of Mother's Day we can see just how incredible it is to think that we have collectively, as a species, decided to dedicate an entire day just to celebrate a parent. The very notion of it is a recognition of just how deep and powerful that connection of mother and child is.

And without a mother, our beautiful babies would never have come to exist at all. So let's take some time to celebrate that. Can you imagine your baby never existing? No, you don't want to, do you? Despite the pain and hurt that comes with their death, the boundless love that comes with their life outweighs it monumentally. Their existence is down to you. No doubt you are already finding ways to honour and remember your baby; this is your legacy of motherhood. Let the day be a celebration of that, of your baby and of YOU.

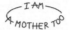

If we want to explore further just how admirable the gift of motherhood is, in all its squiggly and untraditional sittings, then we only have to look around us. Even in the animal realm, we witness the unique connection between mother and child, and of course the bonds between father and child too. We see turtles making great pilgrimages to rest their eggs in safe places, birds carefully taking the time and energy to create nests for their chicks, kangaroos scurrying their young into pouches for warmth and comfort.

And being a mother does not stop if our babies can't stay. We carry with us that nurture and compassion, it is ingrained into our gut, and we invest it into our babies' memory, creating lasting legacies and distributing the love elsewhere. When our babies arrived they came with a parcel, a big box of love, and they left that love with us. Just as any mother's love grows, so does ours. We invest what we can into remembering our own baby and, with the rest of the love, well it's up to us what we do with that. But wouldn't it do our babies a great justice if we sprinkled it around like the gold dust it is, carrying out acts of kindness and saying their names as we do so.

Your baby may not be visible on Mother's Day, but they live on through you, they rely on your actions to nurture their memory.

If you are looking for a proactive way to celebrate this new abundance of love, creating little 'random acts of kindness' parcels to distribute is a really meaningful and fulfilling task. Maybe it is trinkets boxed up and scattered around town, each with a little note telling the lucky discoverer your baby's name and wishing them a peaceful Mother's Day, or decoratively painted pebbles left hidden along popular walking routes. Or perhaps it is a physical act, a monetary or material donation in your baby's name, or even a day volunteering in a homeless shelter or charity close to your heart. With each act of kindness you are distributing love gifted to you by your baby, and you can dedicate the results to them.

You can end the day by saying, 'Thank you baby, you gave me this love and look what I did with it.'

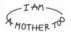

Alongside the more traditional ways of marking the day, such as visiting a memorial with flowers and taking a fresh air walk, you can spend some time sitting with your thoughts, snuggled in bed with your partner or sat in a nursery holding some of your baby's items close to you. You can close your eyes and contemplate just how immense the title of 'mother' is. What a gift, the most admirable and life-changing gift. And who is responsible for this incredible gift? Your baby, of course.

You can really take some time, away from the world, to fill your heart with deep gratitude. You can thank your baby for existing, in whatever form that may be. With thanks to them you have crossed an almighty threshold, you have transformed from 'woman' to 'mother'. It is the greatest title to be crowned with, an absolute honour to know that you are now, and forever will be, a mother.

Would you like a gift? Maybe you would like to begin a memorial in your garden and could take the opportunity of Mother's Day to plant seeds, ready to witness their bloom over the years to come. Or you could request to have your baby's ashes transformed into jewellery. You could choose a photograph keepsake, or simply a bouquet of flowers and a card addressed to 'Mummy'. Be bravely vocal about what you would like and what you want to do, so those around you will be able to meet expectations that they may have otherwise been too nervous to carry out, in fear of upsetting you.

Perhaps you already have other living children. What have all your babies taught you? That a mother's love comes on an endless roll. It does not diminish or wear thin when spread across several offspring. A mother's love simply grows and grows, just when we imagine it has reached its highest height, our love stretches once more beyond sight. More children just equals more love.

Our babies taught us that our hearts have capacity to love beyond bounds. That is powerful lesson and one to thank our babies for.

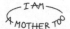

There is no denying that parts of the day will hurt, I'm sure that goes without saying. I remember my first Mother's Day without Winter. Dean bought me flowers to take to the memorial, then we went out for lunch with photographs of our son (and his tiny urn smuggled in Deans pocket ... hey, nothing is weird if it comforts you!). I felt just full of gratitude and love, until a young family with a baby the same age as Winter sat at the table next to us. Naturally, they were celebrating. I felt a lot of warmth for them, but I also experienced a huge rush of pain, and I hid in the toilets in tears before we left.

I share this experience because there is no shame in it. You are always allowed to feel how you feel. You can expect the day to throw challenges, particularly when you see families celebrating what you are simply remembering. You are likely to feel jealous and bitter, your heart can be struck in agony. And you can always remove yourself from anything that bears too great a burden; you can politely turn down an invite that will give rise to too much pain. That's all OK. It doesn't mean the day is a failure, ruined or marred, it just means that you are loving your baby and missing them too. By telling those around you how you would like to spend the day you can set your own expectations.

If celebration feels too far-fetched, then simply marking the day may be enough for you. No matter how deep your grief, you are now undeniably a mother, and this special day has taken on new meaning. Even just a gentle nod to the day is enough. Perhaps your heart is too fragile, perhaps today you turn off social media, close the blinds and squirrel yourself away. Perhaps next year you will feel more able to embrace the day. There is never any right or wrong – if it suits your grief and it doesn't harm others then you are perfectly entitled to do whatever feels right. But don't ever forget that magical bottom line – your baby is loved, there is no doubt about that, and they love you back, of course they do, why wouldn't they? And perhaps that little truth could give rise to a small celebration at least.

You are their mother today and always.

As Mother's Day arrives you can:

* Remember, once a mother always a mother. Take time to relish your title.
* Think how you would like to mark the day, perhaps visiting a special place and creating new special memories.
* Or, find a way to honour your baby, such as random acts of kindness or a donation in their memory.

✳ Tell those close to you what you would like to do, so they can confidently join in your celebration or support you as you hibernate.

✳ Remember that you can allow yourself time to grieve, and the day isn't 'ruined' if you find celebration difficult.

A FESTIVAL OF
FEELING

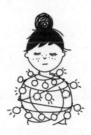

Christmas is inevitably a difficult time – not just for those who have lost a baby, but for anyone who is traipsing through the ravages of grief. It is a time for family, happiness and memory making, all of which can feel like polar opposites to the bereaved's current world. For those of us who are mourning the loss of a child, it is a particularly double-edged sword. After all, Christmas centres so vividly around children, and no doubt we had already excitedly imagined the festive season with that very first positive pregnancy test.

In order to navigate this exceptionally difficult time, I have put together some thoughts and gentle suggestions to help carry you through the festivities.

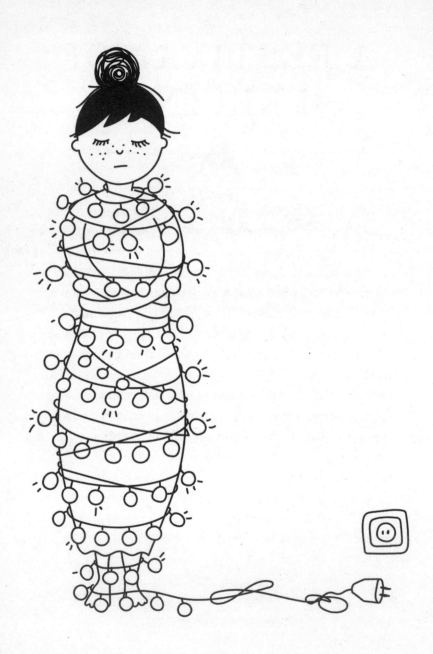

A Festival of Feeling

The first thing to really consider is that Christmas will
happen whether we choose to involve ourselves or not.
Perhaps we may try to cut Christmas altogether from our
lives while our hearts feel too heavy, perhaps we may succeed
in some sort of self-induced hibernation, and perhaps we are
happiest with that decision. But out there, in the big wide
world, all around us, Christmas is still going to happen. The
likelihood that we are able to shield ourselves entirely is very
slim. TV adverts, twinkling lights on the tree outside our
house, Christmas songs on the radio – even holed up at home
in our anti-festive bubble, Christmas makes an uninvited
appearance. To put such effort into neglecting Christmas we
are likely to only invite more misery upon ourselves. And
so, rather than blockade a raging river with a damn made of
sticks, acceptance is the gentlest option for our hearts.

Christmas is coming, the festive season will arrive ... and
pass. Rather than trying to defend ourselves against it with
futile aversion, we can make peace with the fact and instead
decide for ourselves just how we will honour our babies in
the season they are absolutely still a part of – the season of
family.

Something I like to do is imagine myself swapping places
with Winter. If I had died during childbirth and my son
had lived, would I be floating around or sat on a cloud – or
wherever we believe ourselves to reside after death – willing
and wishing my loved ones to have a miserable Christmas?
Would I sit beside them in spirit and hope for them to miss
out on the joys of the season? It's an easy answer, because
we don't ever want to actively wish misery on our loved

ones. What we would hope for is for them to partake in the festivities and embrace the magic, with us in their thoughts.

Guilt is the enemy of bereaved parents. If we allow ourselves to accept and even enjoy Christmas, we can feel the pull of guilt whispering to us, *But you should be sad because your baby died*. The majority of loss families I have spoken to have experienced this, it's a perfectly normal emotion, but when we really consider it we can see that it is absolutely unnecessary to torment ourselves in such a way. During any celebrations where guilt sneaks in, you can remember the bottom line: your baby is loved, they will forever be loved, they know they are loved, nothing in the physical world will ever change any of that. You cannot live your life devoid of any happiness, and certainly your baby – who no doubt loves you back with the same ferocity – would never wish that for you. You love your baby and wherever they are you wish them happiness; your baby loves you and wherever they are they wish you happiness.

Finding some peace and the strength to celebrate Christmas does not equate to you forgetting your baby, it is instead a new opportunity to honour them in a lifelong tradition.

Removing any expectations as to how we think the day *should* go can relieve us of unnecessary pressure. No doubt we had this Christmas set up in our minds already, bump photos by the tree or a baby dressed as a little elf. Realising this will not be the reality stings. Those dreams will not come to fruition and it would be cruel to burden ourselves with a whole new list of expectations.

This Christmas is different from last year, it is a whole new embodiment of the festive season. If we think back over Christmases passed, we will realise that each year our Christmas has been different in some way or other, some ups and some downs. While losing a baby is of course the extreme, we can see that very little in our life goes to plan, and nothing in life ever stays the same.

There is — not now or ever — a way that Christmas should go. Smiles, tears, love, heartbreak, pride, a day littered with memories or an entire day under the duvet, it will go as it goes.

In the beginning, you can just think small. There's no rush to jump right into a Christmas you are not comfortable with. Perhaps spend some time contemplating Christmas, imagining it gently. See the lights springing up, watch its slow descent into stores. Instead of dread and panic, invite in a feeling of acceptance. Christmas is coming and it's OK. Trust that it is survivable.

Putting up the tree is a moment when many people feel they are beginning to embrace the magic. It is the act that says, 'Christmas has officially begun in this home.' Perhaps it feels as though putting a tree up is a big step. I know that it was something I had envisioned doing with a little baby in my arms, and to begin with the thought of putting it up made me feel very hollow. But over time my family have collected many remembrance baubles, and in that sense it feels as though our tree is a festive nod to our baby boy. At a time when there is no baby to buy gifts for, you can ask friends and family to pick up a tree decoration in your baby's memory. Angel wings, initials, name baubles and decorations that hold photographs and handprints, there are many beautiful decorations that can honour our babies. This becomes a great way to begin to feel excited for putting up the tree, as you pick out decorations and gather a special collection. My tree now sits every year blanketed in an ever-growing collection of baubles chosen specifically for our son, and in a sense putting the tree up is the beginning of us including Winter in the festivities.

And you don't need to stop at the tree, you can decorate your whole home with your baby in mind. A miniature Christmas tree can bring a gentle festive touch to the nursery, and twinkling lights can drape over photographs. Christmas-scented candles can be lit next to a hand or footprint, or any other memorial keepsakes. Although it inevitably feels bleak at times, that this is the best we can do, I always take the time to hold my baby in my thoughts with every embellishment, decorating for him, with him.

Christmas brings with it a sense of family togetherness, a feeling that is like a dagger to the heart when our whole idea of family has been pulled apart. But this is still a chance to celebrate the family we do have, and to embrace those who grieve alongside us. You can take a moment to thank your baby for the precious lessons their brief life taught you.

The first lesson, that life is impermanent, it will end one day, and we do not know when that day will be. I like to thank Winter for reminding me that life is such an extraordinarily precious gift and not something that is ever guaranteed from one day to the next. It is something that I always knew, but it wasn't ever a reality. To lose something so precious so swiftly, it is a reminder that those who we love must be loved *right now*. Our babies reminded us that we never really know when life will run out. Christmas is an opportunity to honour your baby by loving those around you with the greatest of gusto.

A second great lesson from our baby is a realisation of just how little meaning material possessions can have. Unless soaked in sentimentality, objects are of less value when you have lost something of such great worth. One carefully chosen and lovingly packaged gift is enough to pass on to your friends and family, and wrapping them up in love is the greatest gift you can give. Our baby taught us about the true value of love above material goods, and in that sense they taught us the true meaning of Christmas.

The third lesson is that our baby taught us about the suffering of others. Once we have experienced such a deep and profound grief, our eyes are inevitably opened to suffering elsewhere in the world. Your baby gave you the gift of new-found compassion and Christmas is the perfect season to put it into practice. I have collected gifts for Winter and gifted them to a local hospital – baby grows, toys and toiletries for parents waiting nervously by their child's bedside. We asked friends and family to buy a little gift 'for Winter' that we could pass on in his memory. It is a way for his life to continue beyond death, with other babies and families benefitting from his very existence.

As we walk the streets we realise that we are carrying such an invisible burden, what other unseen burdens do those around us carry? Our baby gave us the realisation that we all need to be kinder to each other, even to those who aren't kind to us. We never know the torment another person is suffering. During Christmas time, when the town centre is busy and queues are long and tempers are running short, you can honour your baby with this new understanding by sprinkling kindness everywhere you go. Whether you allow someone in a rush to jump the queue or use your spare change to pay for someone's lost parking ticket, you can dedicate this kind act to the baby you love so deeply.

Clever, wise little babies they are.

Aside from buying and donating to charity, there are other ways you can buy for your baby too. We always hang a stocking for our son, but it pains me to see it empty when ours are stuffed with tiny little trinkets. And so I fill it. Just small gifts, a new candle to sit beside his photograph, a new frame for a picture, a little teddy bear, an ornament to decorate his memorial spot. There are some really beautiful online stores now that specialise in baby loss gifts, with imaginative and unique ideas for our babies. Some may also like to buy an item of clothing that would fit their baby now, just to have a sense of their growth and to escape reality for a few moments. If it suits your grief then just do it.

Another way of sharing gifts in our babies' memories is to give gifts with them in mind. A few gifts I have shared in my son's honour include frames that collected feathers can be kept in, with the engraving 'Hello from Winter'. Another time I wrapped a snuggly blanket for my loved ones to cuddle under, with the poem:

Gather together,
get cosy and snug,
and think of me,
when you're wrapped up in love.

Helping to create new cosy memories that are inevitably intertwined with my son's memory; board games, specific films, tickets to a family event, gifts that bring people together, all given with a tag signed from Winter. It's a chance to get a little creative too. If you're crafty then hand-made personalised gifts from your baby are just perfect, such as hand and footprints made into jewellery. And it can be simple and affordable but still super-special. One year I gave out jars with scraps of paper and a poem, to record thoughts of our little boy throughout the year:

Although my life was oh so brief,
I felt the love from you,
so I hatched this little sneaky plan,
to stop you feeling blue,
here you find some paper,
and an empty little jar,
for you to fill with happy thoughts,
while I watch you from afar.
Whenever you feel thankful,
as you go about your day,
think of me your [nephew/grandson],
make a note right away.
Now I can feel peaceful,
that when you climb into bed,
you can dream a special happy dream,
and wear a smile instead.
And so as the year continues,
and my birthday then will come,
we can open up our jar notes,
and share with everyone.

And finally, let's be really kind to ourselves over Christmas, with lots of self-compassion. It is inevitably a raw time of year and we can expect that there will be moments of pain and sadness, moments of tears and certainly moments where we deeply wish it was a different experience altogether. We don't need to suppress any feelings. If something feels too difficult then we just don't do it. Nothing is compulsory, everything is our own decision to make.

Something I like to consider is that my son didn't experience one single Christmas, that experience was stolen from him along with his life. But I am here, experiencing it for yet another year – it's difficult to not see that as privilege. I know Winter would have loved Christmas, and so I will love it for him.

If you can't have Christmas with *your baby, have Christmas* for *your baby.*

So as Christmas arrives you can find ways to celebrate the festive season:

* Gently accept the arrival of Christmas.
* Remove expectations as to how the day should go.
* Remember of all the lessons your baby taught you, the importance of loving your family and friends and offering love and compassion to others who are suffering too.
* Find ways to include your baby in the preparations, such as by collecting remembrance baubles and placing candles by their photos.
* Think of ways to include them in the actual day, too, by giving out gifts in their memory or raising a toast to them over Christmas dinner.

ONE
SWIFT LAP

In the world of living babies, birthdays are a celebration of
achievements and a nostalgic look back over a year filled with
heart-warming memories. In the world of baby loss, birthdays
can feel like a roll call of missed milestones and serve only as
a reminder of the widening gap between your baby's physical
existence and the present day. It is inevitably a bittersweet
event, but with some time and focus it is also possible to find
the energy to wish your baby a happy birthday and maybe
even give them a little (or big) birthday celebration in their
honour. Whether you lost your baby in the womb or after
birth, there is always opportunity to mark the day, whether
you choose to do it privately or publicly.

The run up can panic us, as we inevitably feel there
is a huge amount of pressure on this one day that fast
approaches. For me, it was as though I was being wound up,
each day my chest feeling tighter, my heart just not ready to
accept a year had passed. I imagined the day almost like a
line that was defining of our journey somehow. I was afraid

that it marked the end of something, the end of being freshly bereaved and the world suddenly expecting me to begin moving on.

My anxiety was palpable. We were approaching a finish line but I didn't want to compete in the race. I wanted to push time back, I was desperate to remain in the days that were closest to my baby. As time pulled us apart, I felt the pull physically too. The last time I touched him, kissed him, smelt him, it was all being slowly plucked from my grasp, and I was clinging on to the cliff edge with just my fingertips.

The ongoing heartfelt wish to remain as C L O S E to your baby as possible manifests itself not just in objects and memories, but also in time.

While many of these feelings are universally shared the world over in baby loss, I realised in the end that much of my run-up anxiety was unfounded. As with so many highly charged life events – interviews, first dates, public speaking – our imagination has a tendency to run away into the most exaggerated possibilities. Such high emotional expectations, the feeling that all our intense grief will rise to the surface and explode. But in reality, the day arrives as any other, filled with sadness, yes, but also presenting an opportunity to include our baby in a day that will forever be special to us.

For many in the loss community, our baby's birthday is also an anniversary of their death. Birth and death, events which should be separated by years and experiences, instead compounded into one single day. Other times our wombs cradled our babes so gently to sleep and kept them safe and close for days or weeks before we physically birthed them. Death before birth is so painfully topsy turvy in its nature, but regardless of this tragic circumstance, the day our baby was delivered earth side remains to be a poignant and life changing moment. The day they 'arrived', their day of birth. On this special day that commemorates their entrance into the world, we can allow ourselves both the space to grieve and the space to celebrate. And we can remember that death is only able to happen where life first flourished, and their life is forever bigger than their death. As we grieve their loss of life and their stolen opportunities, we can also celebrate the very fact that they exist, they are real, they are important and they are loved. Whether with or without breath, they were birthed from womb to Earth and therefore still achieved this day to commemorate.

We have this new date etched into our calendar forever – a date that they brought to our attention so vividly, a date that without their existence would have passed us by without much notice, a date that has therefore become special. A birthday is an opportunity for us to reflect on the year that has passed, and smoke out the better memories among the difficult ones. You can reflect on your journey and any precious moments you shared with your baby, along with all the spectacular lessons their brief life has taught you. You can realise just how much of a privilege it is to be alive to celebrate a birthday, and how fortunate you are to grow older, and this can give you added motivation to make something special of theirs.

As the day looms over the horizon, you can take a moment to decide, *How will I spend this special day?* As with anything in this world of baby loss, there is no right or wrong way to invest your time, you just have to find what is going to suit you best. Would you like to spend the day with your partner and take a fresh air walk as you talk about your baby? Or would you like to gather with family at your baby's memorial spot? While some people may feel that it is just too painful to have a cake with no one to blow out the candles and choose to steer well clear of an open celebration, others may decide they want to mark the day in the more traditional way with a real-life party, and either is absolutely a valid choice. Whatever you decide, taking the time to think it through in advance gives you the chance to set plans in place and relieve a little of the uncertainty around the day.

If you do decide to keep the day just for yourself and your partner and your other children, there are many options to keep your intimate gathering special. The planting of a flower or tree in your garden, a visit to somewhere memorable from your pregnancy, or a quiet meal together with the opportunity to talk and remember your baby. The day is yours to do with what you wish – it is an open book, one you can write however suits you best.

If you decide to have a bigger celebration, then there's no reason why you can't. A party without the main guest may seem unusual, but why not? A child, whether in your arms or in your heart, is deserving of whatever you decide is appropriate. Dean and I chose to have a huge party for our son's first birthday, and the busy and uplifting nature of the day was exactly what my heart required.

The very idea of a birthday party may seem unconventional, but then so is your experience of motherhood. You can embrace that and say, 'We want to have a party, so we will!'

Perhaps you will choose to have the celebration at your home and keep just close friends and family on the invites, or perhaps you will decide to create something much bigger. With this in mind you could take the opportunity to involve the community if you wish and create a fundraising celebration. We can be brave and spread the word on social media, call the local newspaper, ask friends and family to bake cakes to bring along and then display them on a table with a donation pot in exchange for a slice.

Often you will have something that reminds you of your baby, such as a star or a butterfly, and these are a perfect basis for a light theme. This also gives you the chance to spend the lead up to the birthday making special preparations, such as themed table decorations or bunting, which offers a peaceful distraction and gentle meaning in these approaching days.

From my own experience of early miscarriage, I know that a birthday is not always the most obvious date. A birthday can instead stretch across many days, from the date that we sadly lost our baby to the date they were due to be birthed. Marking the birthday of an earlier loss can offer its own challenges. The more private or possibly secret nature of such loss can make the date feel quite lonely; it feels brushed aside by those around us who cannot fathom the potential magnitude of the day. For each early loss I have experienced, the due dates have always remained etched into my memory, and the dates that I lost those babies are also something I will never forget.

You may find that friends and family are deeply encouraging in your intentions to mark the significant days, but you may also be made to feel as though you are somehow over-egging it. As parents to a baby, no matter how brief their life, you can always remain assured that you are entitled to celebrate or grieve on these days however you wish. You can see this as another opportunity to gently educate those around you of the world of baby loss and its enduring impact on our lives. These are days that will forever hold the 'what ifs' and 'could have beens'. They are dates that changed your life and introduced you to both a pain and love that you were yet to know. They are dates that deserve marking in some way even if it is simply the lighting of a candle or holding your baby extra close in your thoughts.

However we decide to mark our baby's birthday, we can be certain of one thing – their very existence is worthy of recognising and celebrating.

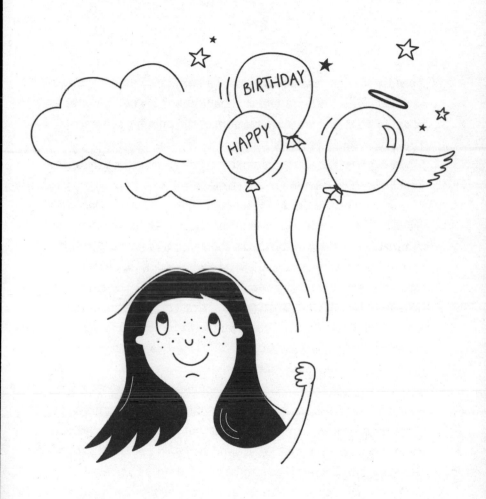

Once the day has passed, there is the familiar feeling of calm after the storm. We can feel as though there is a new chapter about to start, but we are uncertain of the opening sentence. There is so much emphasis on the big day that the days following can lead us back into feeling like a lost sheep. *Now what?!* One birthday down, a lifetime to go.

As we take the time to gather ourselves once more, we realise we are facing a forever without our baby. Such is the significance of the first birthday, the passing of it leads us into further unknowns. Personally, I struggled much more with my son's second birthday than his first, feeling as though the novelty of his life and death was wearing thin to those around me and his memory was fading farther from my reach. A sense of, *Another birthday passed and so many more to come*, left me feeling floored and emotional.

The ongoing fight to keep our baby present in the memories of those around us can be exhausting and lonely. In these moments we can be reminded that grief rules our heart these days, and that's OK, that's the way it will be. Your baby will always and forever be special and present to you and those who care about them. Birthdays are always going to be a challenge, our grief will fluctuate and that is to be expected. And what I really want to say is, don't be frightened.

The passing of time can feel so very cruel as you grieve the loss of your baby, and birthdays can feel like an unbearable hurdle. But my own experience taught me to not be afraid. The day itself can be remarkably peaceful, a whole day in fact that is dedicated to the memory of your baby, surrounded by friends and family and blanketed in love. If we remove expectations and the pressure of what *must be* then we find we have an opportunity to honour our baby and show them just how much they mean to us. Of course there is grief muddled in, sadness and heartbreak and the desperate wish for what we should have had, our baby is important and they deserve our tears. This day does not mark the end of your grief, it simply marks the continuation of your love.

I once heard a description for the meaning of 'time' that has forever stayed with me: 'Time is a perimeter that measures change'. That is all it is, and while things change around us – the seasons, our home, our skin – the love for our babies remains forever enduring. As humans with an organising nature, we have titled 'time' and categorised it into neat calendars. Three hundred and sixty-five days, one whole year, one swift lap of the Earth around our beaming sun. The movements of the universe have offered us these markers without regard for our hearts, and we gather them and title them, and at times we cower at the expectations they present to us. But one whole year is simply time passing with a name – 365 days and we miss our babies, but we miss them at 369 days, we miss them at 300 days and we will miss them still at 400. The big scary ONE YEAR mark is really just as big and scary – and survivable – as any other daily, weekly or monthly mark we endure in the endless run of life after baby loss. My fear that my baby's birthday would mark the end of something was entirely unfounded. It wasn't the end, there was no grand finale. And the same goes for you.

Your story is not yet finished. It does not finish at loss, it does not finish at a first-year anniversary, and it will not finish even if you go on to have other children.

As your baby's birthday approaches you can:

❋ Expect to feel anxious and overwhelmed in the run up.
❋ Ease some of that anxiety by deciding how you would like to spend the day and beginning to put some plans in place.
❋ Plan a big party, a small family gathering or time alone with your partner.
❋ Allow yourself time to both grieve and celebrate, and remove the pressure of expectation.
❋ Remember time can never separate you from the love and memories you hold for your baby.

IMPATIENTLY WAITING

I remember vividly a conversation with a bereavement midwife shortly after we lost our son, where I 'admitted' that I was desperate to start trying for another baby right away. It felt like an admission, because really I believed, like many others who experience the loss of a baby, that I should wait for a bit. But wait for what, I don't know. For grief to end? To be over the death of my son? Moments that, of course, would never come. The bereavement midwife, recognising my timid guilt, smiled and said, 'Typically when a baby dies people fall into two categories. Either they cannot ever imagine themselves ever wanting another baby, or they want to begin trying again right away.'

Trying to conceive following a loss is a personal journey that varies so drastically from person to person. While some become pregnant so quickly, for others the road is longer and bumpier, but the general consensus is shared – it is P A I N S T A K I N G. It took me and my partner fourteen months and two miscarriages to finally get the positive test that resulted in our rainbow baby. Fourteen months felt like a lifetime. And yet I'm all too aware of how fortunate we were, and how our time trying was just a mere drop in the ocean compared to many families who try for years to be pregnant and bring home a baby.

Trying to conceive harboured some of my saddest and darkest moments. It is an unbearable weight to add to the burden of grief, and with no promised finished line it could leave me feeling hopeless.

Even for someone who excels at finding the positives in dire situations, I struggled to make light work of trying to conceive. It is a tremendously difficult and emotionally fraught time. And so forgive me if this chapter feels particularly heavy and bleak, but I'm hoping that by simply sharing my own experience as honestly and as rawly as possible, we can all understand how challenging it is and just how normal our feelings can be during this time.

My personal journey of trying to conceive went something like this. When we first decided to try for a baby, the word 'try' was pretty much null and void. I took my last contraceptive pill on Christmas Day and I was six weeks pregnant before I even considered taking a pregnancy test just two months later. Like many people who conceive quickly, I had no idea of just how fortunate I had been. By October our son arrived, and died. And trying to conceive would never be the same again.

I naively imagined myself falling pregnant again right away and bringing home another baby before my son's first anniversary. Little did I know my days of casually 'trying' and happily peeing onto a positive test were so far behind me. I was stepping into entirely new territory.

What began with optimism and enthusiasm quickly became an obsession of dates and timings and a life lived cycle to cycle, and there is nothing like the pure desperation for a life after loss to steal any fun out of baby making. Something so intimate and personal, once so relaxed and carefree, is soon an essential and well-timed task that is imperative in the making of ALL our hopes and dreams. The end goal has changed; it is no longer a small, fun part of the relationship puzzle, instead it fast becomes a huge deal and can even shift long-standing relationship dynamics.

It begins with the desperation for the golden 'fertility window', when it seems as though everything is at stake. Four days or so that hold your whole future to ransom – the pressure that comes with that knowledge is intense. After younger years spent trying to avoid getting pregnant at all costs, suddenly the chances of it actually happening seem entirely minuscule. It is impossible to not end up working out your odds, a handful of possible days, percentage chances that you time it right and sperm actually does meet the egg, just 13 cycles in a year. I experienced a huge rush of anxiety and an overwhelming sense of time running out during those days which, let's be honest, hardly makes for the most relaxed and romantic intimate moments. There is an almighty feeling of 'now or never', a real desperate scramble to 'catch the egg'. During those days, and the run up, my chest felt constantly tight with anticipation, the urgency and drive to always give ourselves the best chance was consuming. So much rested on it, the fierce desire to fill my womb, and subsequently my arms, was so deeply engrained in me I could not bear the thought of another month passing by wasted.

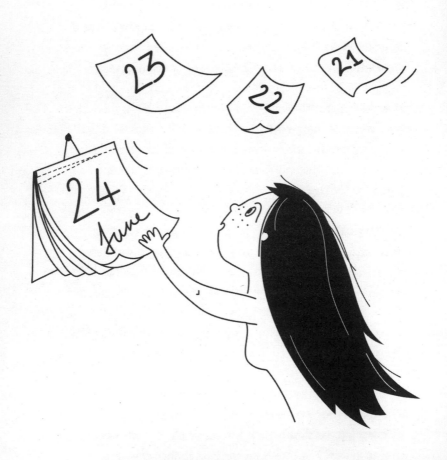

Once the fertile window draws to a close, the dreaded 'two week wait' begins. The mental torture inflicted by the waiting feels unbearable. On the one hand we are wishing the time away, clawing at the next fortnight to see if our efforts brought the reward we so longed for, on the other hand each week pulls us further away from the time we spent with our lost baby.

Trying to conceive after loss is a real tug of war of emotions, constantly stuck between wishing time away and willing it to slow down.

It is a crushing space to sit in, to never feel relaxed enough to accept the current moment, instead always feeling torn between two worlds – our past and our future. There is the obsessive questioning: 'Did we do enough?' 'Did we get the timings right?' 'Is this our month?' And of course: 'Is it too early to test?' After scouring online sites for early pregnancy symptoms I almost always caved and tested far too early, resulting in a negative test that left me heartbroken and consumed by hopelessness and grief. And yet still I believed that somehow I had been too keen to test and maybe, possibly, hopefully those two lines would show themselves tonight, tomorrow, later in the week.

I could always pinpoint what would be my due date had we been successful, and it was near on impossible to not let my aching imagination catch fire. A baby in time for Christmas, a baby arriving for spring, a summer baby. I became so lost in my own world, constantly holding my breath, constantly tense, constantly knotted stomach. The temptation to put *everything else* on hold. It was as though I couldn't move forward or even dare to make plans. I didn't want to book the holiday, just in case I was pregnant, and I was afraid to make plans away from my partner in case it fell during my fertile window. So determined and so frightened, I lived within a tunnel, avoiding anything that I believed, rightly or wrongly, could damage my chances in any way. My whole life centred around dates and one desperate wish.

And then it came, the unwanted period. Even with early spotting I clung on to hope that it was implantation bleeding. I sat reading stories online of women who still had periods even when pregnant. But the time came when it was no longer deniable, and each and every time I felt floored by grief and heartbreak. I sobbed and sobbed, so entirely unable to cope with the truth that my arms were to remain empty yet again.

I was pulled from my distracted and hopeful imaginary world and thrown straight back into the reality that my baby had died.

It is during this stage that we can find it particularly difficult to listen to other people's advice or opinions, and almost impossible to reason with facts. I was always unable to step outside my own bubble and see things clearly. I was so engrossed in the end goal that words of support felt empty, no matter how love-filled they were. The statement that I should 'Just relax and it will happen' was not enough for me. I needed more, I needed to know that it would definitely beyond doubt happen. I needed confirmation from somewhere, anywhere. Comments that 'You've been pregnant before so you must be able to get pregnant again' fell quite rightly on deaf ears. It was too late for me then – I knew the truth, I knew that secondary infertility was a thing. I knew that some women were only ever blessed with one child, and I wondered with great pain if Winter had been my one and only chance.

It was an incredibly lonely time, and so difficult for friends and family to truly grasp the level of desperation pinned on each and every cycle. I was aware that no one could really help me. My one wish rested on something that was ultimately so invisible and impossible to touch or physically manipulate, so entirely out of my control. I relied mostly on online forums and found comfort in other 'trying to conceive' accounts on Instagram. There I discovered a whole world of other women who were feeling exactly how I felt and I found my emotions were validated. I wasn't going crazy, I was just experiencing the messy and crushing world of trying to conceive after loss, and it was as hard as hell.

Fertility is still a hushed topic and there is some level of shameful feelings when we are unable to become pregnant or keep a pregnancy. We feel, unjustly, that the fault lies with us. As a woman armed with a womb but unable to put it to use, we feel broken, we feel ashamed, we feel incomplete.

So hushed is the topic that many women are not educated in their cycles – I find it difficult to believe I was the only woman with such little knowledge of my own insides. It was only when I failed to fall pregnant as quickly as I did with my first baby that I began to look deeper into the workings of my body. I was surprised at my stark lack of basic understanding, my life previous to this point had simply never required me to learn the more intricate rhythms of a monthly cycle.

The discovery of the four-day window was a win/lose situation. It both improved our chances and heightened the anxiety. It came with a sense of empowerment, but the price tag was knowledge of the two week wait. While I found this new-found information helpful, at times I clung to it so tightly that it was suffocating. It is a such a fine line to tread. I armed myself with ovulation sticks and cycle tracking apps, convinced I needed them for the ultimate chance, but I often became disenchanted, removing myself from the dastardly circle of hope, desperation and grief by throwing the sticks in the bin and deleting the fertility app. Inevitably I returned to them, sheepishly, and the obsession sank back in, but then a moment of liberation and attempting to relax I once again deleted the calendars and binned the sticks. Up and down, up and down. Trying to conceive after loss isn't so much a roller coaster, it is much more like a hike up and down a mountain. It's a slog that continues until we one day, hopefully, via whatever means necessary, become pregnant and begin the journey to our much-wanted baby.

Trying to conceive following loss is one hell of a journey. It is lonely, painful and desperate. With the gift of hindsight, from my own personal experience, I can offer the following guidance:

* Recognise the wibbly-wobbly journey ahead of you; know it may not be smooth and simple. Expect a tornado of emotions, brace yourself and, above all, know it will be worth it in the end.
* Read up, educate yourself on your cycle and each monthly opportunity. Empower yourself with information.
* Try not to let obsession engulf you. It's likely to peak and trough, so just go with however you are feeling, but try to give yourself a break from the sticks and charts from time to time.
* Continue to live! Don't put everything else on hold. Easier said than done, I didn't manage it, but I hope you do – either way, just try.
* Find your tribe. Join support groups and connect with others in a similar situation. Instagram has a huge community – search the #ttc hashtag. Reach out to friends, share your journey.
* Where possible, talk to your loved ones in open conversation, tell them how difficult this path truly is.

GROWING HOPE

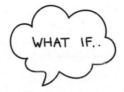

After the debilitating trauma of baby loss, the endless slog of grief and the psychological torture of trying to conceive, a positive test could feel like a welcome relief. But pregnancy after loss, although worth celebrating, brings with it its own challenges. So here are some survival tips and food for thought to help you navigate the next colossal hurdle in your journey to take home a living baby.

The very first thing you can do is to accept that the pregnancy you are embarking on is going to be a different experience to your previous pre-loss pregnancy. Although you may have been aware that some pregnancies end in loss, until we experience loss ourselves we can remain incredibly naive to it, believing that as we are healthy and living in a wealthy country with abundant healthcare, there is very little reason to worry. If we have been fortunate enough to have a smooth and gentle pregnancy prior to loss, full of happy memories and excited preparations, then these are moments we can hold in our heart and keep in our bank of precious memories, but these moments are unlikely to be replicated so easily in any future pregnancies.

Pregnancy after loss is a vastly different experience; it is a NEW experience. Take some time to sit with that thought, then let go of expectations and embrace the new journey that lies before you.

Regular pregnancy experiences such as scans and baby preparation take on a whole new surreal edge. I remember being nothing but excited to see my baby on a screen during my first pregnancy, but once pregnant with my daughter I would sit in the waiting room with a stomach full of knots and a lingering sense of doomsday dread. For days leading up to a scan, my anxiety would slowly rise as my racing mind imagined a long line of catastrophic outcomes. By the time the scan came I was terrified, each hospital check-up felt make or break. When all went well I imagined I was in a computer game and hitting the save button at every visit, *Baby is safe up until now, you may enter the next level.*

What was once full of joyful anticipation is now much more serious and anxiety driven. To help you navigate such immensely poignant milestones such as hospital check-ups, buying rompers, decorating the nursery and baby showers, reach out to those around you and say, 'This isn't an easy moment for me. This is hard, I'm scared.'

You can give yourself time to take stock of how far you have come. You can give yourself time to breathe, eyes closed, hand on belly, 'Today my baby is alive and healthy.'

From my own experience I recognise that there is little that we can do to relieve our racing mind. Words of comfort and strength are greatly received, yet often float in one ear and out the other. When we are so tightly bound to the realisation that everything could end, it is incredibly difficult to move ourselves away from that mindset. By simply allowing yourself to feel frightened you can remove some pressure. If you don't want a baby shower then that's OK. If you can't decorate a nursery then that's OK. If you can't bear to buy a romper in case it is left forever unfilled, then that's OK. In this pregnancy you can live day to day, quite literally taking baby steps. And the moment you feel as though you can indulge in a little preparation, when you make *your own* decision to purchase a tiny pair of socks – and you feel so full of brazen courage, as though you have just leapt over a raging river – you can absolutely allow yourself to celebrate that.

In those moments that are so thieved of naive joy, it is easy to slip into a mindset bitter at those around us who are breezing through a carefree pregnancy. But focusing on what we feel cheated out of is only going to harvest resentment and steal any personal happiness. When scrolling through online sites or preparing ourselves for a scan, we imagine the nonchalant vibe of those fellow pregnant families around us, all revelling in sheer excitement. It's as though we are surrounded by women celebrating so flamboyantly and carefree, sitting with wombs that had never yet betrayed them. And we can feel incredibly alone.

But to those around you, you too are a mother embarking gleefully on the next phase of your life – our painful past like an invisible cloak. And it is the same wherever you go about in your day-to-day life. No one could tell from a glance that you are grieving the loss of your baby; we can never know someone's past – and certainly not their destined future – just by their appearance. As we sit in that waiting room, or read the posts on social sites, we can remember that others are likely to be suffering in other ways, or have experienced suffering in the past. We know now that one in four pregnancies end in loss and those around us are just as vulnerable.

We can wish for those who are about to receive good news for them to immerse themselves vibrantly in their pregnancy, and for those who will receive bad news – either now or later on – to have the most gentlest of journeys possible.

Rather than fester in any bitterness, we can instead recall previous carefree journeys of our own and remember just how special it was. We never wanted to be robbed of that, and therefore we would not want to rob others of it. Instead of thinking, *It's easy for you for, you haven't lost a baby*, it brings us much more peace to accept that other people's experiences are entirely separate to our own, and to instead think, *I wish for you to have a long and healthy pregnancy.*

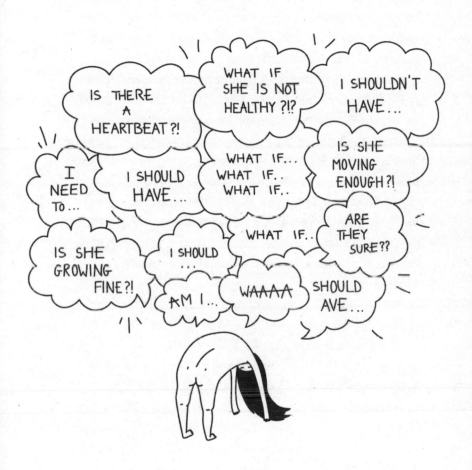

When carrying your new baby, inevitably there is the ongoing fear that the pregnancy will end. It is a fear that can stop us from celebrating the pregnancy altogether. In the beginning I had this nagging sense that the moment I celebrated, that would be when my baby died. Of course, this whole idea may seem unreasonable to someone free from such devastation, but, for me, after my son dying so cruelly and unexpectedly, suffering miscarriages just as we had allowed hope to creep in, I worried that if I dared to celebrate then this would give rise to another cruel repercussion. In some ways I felt undeserving. It's a feeling that is difficult to explain to others, but it was like a little voice saying, *Don't be stupid, this baby won't live, don't be foolish enough to celebrate.* It felt as though I was always going to run out of luck at some point and I would be an idiot to not prepare myself for that moment.

But over time I realised that this way of thinking was stealing any positive experience from the pregnancy. What began as a feeling of self-protection, quickly moved more towards self-punishment, and I ultimately came to understand is that there no such thing as jinxing a pregnancy. Whether you celebrate or not, this will not decide your baby's fate.

I can give the example of my own experiences to cement this point. Three pregnancies that all ended in loss. The first, a smooth and vibrant experience, problem-free, ethereal, full of celebration and excitement, that eventually ended with the healthy birth of my son and his subsequent death the following day. The second, so brief but so full of hope, we were so happy we shared our expectant news with family on Father's Day, only to then lose the baby the day after. And the third, the most delicate pregnancy, where I declined a photograph from the scan for fear of becoming too attached to my growing hope, and I lay as still as a stone on the sofa for weeks just begging the baby to stay safely in my womb, only to miscarry the day before our second scan. All pregnancies were celebrated at differing levels, and all ended in loss. I can draw from these vastly different experiences the knowledge that, whether we hide away and decline an image or throw a shower and frame the scan picture, the outcome is still entirely out of our hands.

So yes, celebrate in any way you can. Take the growing bump photographs, document the kicks and rolls, you can allow yourself to immerse and believe. There is simply no such thing as investing in a pregnancy so much that it will end.

Nothing can end your baby's life except the course of life itself.

For me, at a time when I have so few memories of my son alive, and the majority of those are of him unwell and dying, I count my pregnancy memories as among some of my most cherished. Even those pregnancies that were so incredibly brief held memories of happiness that deserve recognition. When we now understand how brief life can be and how it can cease at any moment, we can also understand that every second counts as life, whether that is in your arms or in your womb.

And yes, it is not easy. It takes strength, huge strength, to celebrate a pregnancy after loss, and there is likely to always be a sense of doubt playing as a constant background noise. It is absolutely reasonable to feel that way. Once we have lived through such a dark trauma we are understandably looking to protect our heart and we are inevitably pulled to our most painful memories. It isn't exactly possible to skip through a post-loss pregnancy, and even with positive focus we are destined to deal with some level of anxiety.

Friends and family around us may not understand our new, less optimistic stance on our pregnancy. Those around me wondered why I still worried endlessly during my daughter's pregnancy. Once we have the deep understanding that a pregnancy – no matter how problem-free and smooth – can end in broken dreams and an empty nursery, there is no going back from that. As with any of these difficult challenges on our journey, our greatest option is to always open up to those close to us. To say, 'I'm happy that I'm pregnant, but I can't always relax and just be optimistic,' is completely OK. If people buy you gifts and you aren't yet ready, then you can thank them, fold the clothes and store them in a cupboard out of sight. You are not being negative or purposely pulling a black cloud over the experience, you are just living through a pregnancy with an explosive wake-up call.

'Is this your first? How many children do you have?'

A simple passing question that I once so relished answering quickly became an anxiety riddled bombshell that I avoided like the plague. When I carried Winter, I *wished* for people to ask me. My swelling belly invited strangers to join in my journey. Anyone who asked this question became witness to my transition into motherhood. 'Yes, my very first baby!' I felt giddy, bashful and full of pride to include anyone and everyone in my first steps to motherhood. But now, my stomach knotted up, my shoulders tensed, even my physical body felt the emotional blow of such a simple question.

The first time I was asked I was unprepared. Only a tiny little bump rested below my ribs, I wasn't ready for anyone I didn't directly know to take great notice. So my suggestion here is to take time early on to think how to answer this question, that way it is a smoother experience for you and the other unknowing party. How you choose to answer is deeply personal and it is *your* choice, there is no rule book as to what you *should* say. The differing experiences of miscarriage, stillbirth and neonatal loss, how you choose to remember your baby and whether you choose to keep your baby private or speak publicly about them, are all valid factors in how you choose to respond.

You may want to acknowledge your previous baby but find the words difficult and the moment too emotional. It can be easier to say, 'Yes this is my first', and if that is what you would prefer to say then there is nothing wrong with it. No, you are not letting down the baby you lost by erasing their memory, you are just making the decision to keep some traumatic and intimate information to yourself.

I role-played this question by myself many times. It's surprising just how many people ask upon seeing a baby bump, so I felt like I needed to be prepared. I found that it was comfortable for me to reply with, 'It's my second baby,' in recognition of my son, and this was usually enough information to satisfy the observer. While I was never internally dismissive of my early miscarriages, I chose to quietly remember those losses – not through shame or embarrassment, but simply my own personal choice. You are absolutely allowed to remember and acknowledge your own losses however feels most peaceful to you.

If the question was followed up with, 'You're going to have your hands full then,' I chose to just smile and say, 'Hopefully.'

If the conversation continued to, 'How old is your other child?', that is when I said something along the lines of, 'Sadly our first baby died. We are looking forward to meeting his brother or sister,' and smiled and gave my belly a rub.

From experience, I found that replying with less direct answers, such as 'My other baby lives in my heart' or 'We didn't get to keep our other baby' meant it was sometimes not clear that Winter had died, and I would then find myself explaining that later on, which gave rise to some uncomfortable realisations from the poor stranger on the bus/ in the shop queue or wherever I happened to be. I also found that ending it on a more positive note gave the other person an easier time deciding what to say next, as I was offering two threads of potential follow-up conversation. They could either acknowledge that my son died or make a comment about being excited to meet our next baby – 'Is it a girl or a boy?', etc. It felt like a gentle way of delivering an emotional blow, which doesn't make the passing stranger feel unnecessarily uncomfortable – because while we live daily with that uncomfortable knowledge that our baby died, it is a deeply sad event and in all honesty not everyone we meet is emotionally prepared to navigate such a devastating fact when it is sprung on them. It isn't hiding it or putting others' feelings first, I think it is more a 'judge your audience' situation. I didn't divulge all to the 16-year-old cashier at Topshop but I did open my heart to the talkative kind lady I sat next to on the bus for 20 minutes.

There may be feelings of guilt that cloud this pregnancy. I often looked at photographs of my son and felt guilty that I was giving life to another baby when I could not give that to him. I felt guilty that I could be fulfilling all the dreams I had for my son, but with another baby. And I felt guilty that I would not be able to spend as much time on his memory as I would inevitably be juggling maintaining his legacy with the demands of raising another child. But we can always remind ourselves of the bottom line that saved me so many times during guilt-drenched moments: we love the babies we have lost, they know they are loved and they love you back, why wouldn't they? And when you love someone you want them to be happy. We can imagine our baby, wherever we believe them to be, watching us, surrounding us, loving us back, and willing us to be happy.

Pregnancy after loss is both challenging and wonderful. The distinct but misplaced feeling that your body failed before and could fail again is terrifying and holds your entire pregnancy to ransom. Our bump grows alongside our knowledge that nothing is guaranteed.

Healthy, live babies are born all day, every day, all over the world; it is entirely possible that your baby will be too.

When treading the tightrope of pregnancy after loss, you can try to:

* Remove expectations and prepare yourself for a new and different pregnancy experience.
* Take this pregnancy one day at a time.
* Tell those around you why it is a challenge. You are not being negative, you are communicating just how complex this journey is.

* Allow yourself to *feel*. Hospital appointments are nerve-racking, being around other pregnant women is hard. It's OK to be afraid, it's OK to find things difficult, it's *normal*. Just don't let it swallow you whole.

* And allow yourself to believe and to celebrate. There is no such thing as jinxing your pregnancy. Enjoy what you can.

* And alongside all of the above, remember that if there is any change in your baby's movements, and anytime you feel that something is wrong, you can call your midwife team and get checked up. Never feel as though you are a burden, never feel as though you are overreacting, simply put yourself and your baby's health first.

THE RAINBOW
AFTER THE
STORM

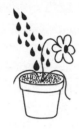

A rainbow baby is the name given to a baby that is born following the loss of a previous baby due to miscarriage, stillbirth or neonatal death. This term is given to these babies as a bright rainbow typically follows a devastating storm, giving us hope and inviting new light into our lives. The term also lovingly recognises that there is no rainbow without a storm, therefore acknowledging the lives of the babies we lost.

So here you are, a rainbow in your arms. And when your longed-for baby arrives you are nothing but happy, your heart is fixed and your grief ends. Right? Of course not. While there are undoubtable highs in the appearance of such a longed-for baby, there are also the endless complexities attached to their arrival. Steering your boat among the debris and learning to celebrate your new life is at times a challenge and, again, those around you may not understand the new-found pain that sits alongside your happiness. New hurdles await, but also too does a whole new world of love.

Firstly, of course it is impossible to have your new baby handed to you and not remember the baby you have lost. Your new baby was brought to existence by the same creators, their beginnings were sparked in the same womb and they were housed in the same human body. The bond they share runs so incredibly deep, so much common ground before breath is even taken. And once born, your rainbow baby is two juxtaposing things: a little delicious slice of your lost baby and their very own individual person. And it's OK, they can be both of these things in harmonious synchronicity. Recognising that they remind us of our lost baby – whether in appearance or simply because of the in-womb bond they share – isn't a sign that we are 'stuck in the past' or longing 'too hard' for a baby we could not keep, it is something much more beautiful than that. It is the realisation that they are family. Siblings that may never physically meet, but will always share DNA and a cord invisible to the naked eye. We can absolutely compare and celebrate the similarities of both of our babies, just as we would have had they both lived.

It is not unhealthy to dust your rainbow in memories of what you lost. In fact it is healthy to see those memories revived and brought to life in all the glorious realness of your rainbow.

Of course it is not easy. While our rainbow baby's arrival brings with it immense happiness, it also invites a new intense round of grief. Looking back over my own journey I can see that a big part of me had hoped for some solace to come with my daughter's arrival. I wasn't prepared to face another fresh blast of grief while navigating the beautiful and overwhelming life-changing bedlam that a newborn brings. I was certainly guilty at some points in my pre-rainbow days of believing that mothers who were lucky enough to have their rainbow babies were somehow a little more healed, and perhaps free from some of the pain inflicted by their previous baby's death. Once Raven arrived, I quickly concluded that this belief was vastly misplaced.

Whether we already have other living children or go on to have a rainbow, there is no alternative circumstance that offers a true remedy from the grief of baby loss. Rainbow babies bring joy and invite fresh meaning into our lives. They are to be celebrated and there is, without a doubt, a whole new injection of love in our veins. But yes, we still hurt from our loss, nothing ever erases that. Happiness and heartbreak simply co-exist.

Amid the pure celebration for our new baby, this renewed grief can leave us utterly blindsided. Birthing a baby creates chaos in our hormones regardless of previous loss, and as bereaved mothers we are left juggling ever more bountiful heightened emotions. We can absolutely recognise that among the joy our rainbow baby brings, we are still allowed to grieve. Our sadness doesn't just evaporate at the arrival of a new baby, our grief simply enters a new dimension, and as our outer lives change our inner feelings are left to play catch up.

With family comes a sense of togetherness and when we have lost a baby we live with the realisation that we will never all be altogether, at least not in the physical sense. While we may already *know* this, when we are finally confronted with the reality it can come as a huge blow. With a new baby's starkly physical presence, we feel as though we can only continue to remember and imagine the baby we lost. It can feel very much as though we are leaving them behind in some way, entering another life without them by our side.

What you can remember in these moments is that your lost baby exists exactly how you choose to envision them. Cast aside they are not; forgotten and in the past they will never be. We know that and we *choose* that. We choose to carry them into the future with us and that is where they will continue to exist. What we have is an opportunity to not only continue our grief for them, but the chance to love them outside the walls of imagination. Your lost baby exists not only in the past, but right here in the present, right in front of our eyes, in touching distance, in the form of a rainbow they are eternally connected to. A living baby awaiting love and affection, entirely dependent upon you, and you are here, completely able to lavish them in enough love for B O T H your babies. It is a chance to act on the love that you have, until now, been forced to play out in other unconventional ways.

And the baby you lost remains with you not only through the physicality of your rainbow, but forever in your heart and mind. Your love and memories are mobile and fluid. They do not remain historical and boxed up, instead you carry them with you through every single present moment. As you make new memories with your rainbow, your love and any memories of your lost baby are not pushed out and replaced, they simply sit alongside them, gathering greater embellishment. Memories simply flex and stretch to include the whole family.

The physical 'altogetherness' may never be, but there is nothing in this earthly world that can emotionally separate a mother and her baby.

I also soon realised that with my daughter I have another person to share my son with, and as she grows up I'm watching him grow up. She's like a sisterly clue as to what Winter could have been. And while it can be difficult to find the time to grieve when parenting an around-the-clock baby, we can all find ways to include our lost baby in our everyday life. For example, I look at Winter's photograph every day as I head downstairs for breakfast, and, with Raven in my arms, we wave and say aloud, 'Good morning Winter.'

There are countless ways you can include your lost baby like this in routine family life. Maybe you have an area of the garden dedicated to your baby and your little rainbow can help to plant seeds and water them. Maybe you light a candle next to a photograph and your rainbow has the honourable job of blowing it out each night, or perhaps there's a teddy bear they can cuddle that sends hugs to their sibling. And bigger future family celebrations can include both babies too. One special egg to find amidst the Easter hunt with your lost baby's symbol or colour. Little hands helping to decorating the Christmas tree with all your baby's special baubles. And perhaps your rainbow could help to bake a birthday cake for your lost baby, or choose flowers to take to a memorial.

Sharing both of your babies together like this also helps to eliminate that nagging guilt that continually comes with life after baby loss. It keeps your lost baby involved and forever a part of the family. And yes, do not ever forget that magical bottom line: your lost baby is loved, you love them, and they love you, of course they do, why wouldn't they? And therefore they wish for you to be happy, and you are allowed to feel happiness with your rainbow. I know I will be telling Raven all about her brother. In my experience children happily accept the reality they are presented with, and sharing the love for our lost babies with them is not morbid or frightening, it simply teaches love without bounds, as we pass on all those lessons we were so generously gifted.

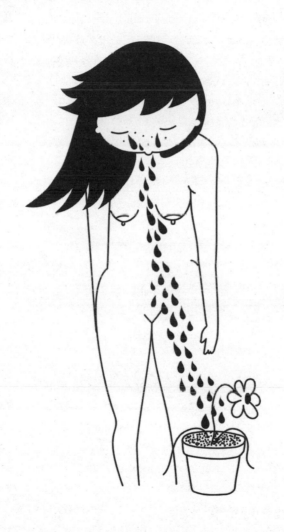

Watching your rainbow grow and learn, you may feel constantly torn in two. With each milestone that your baby reaches, your heart is pulled in opposing directions. Pride, love, happiness and a deep undercurrent of sadness. We are thrilled when our baby giggles for the first time, or masters their roll, and there are so many firsts – first bath, first tooth and first steps. And there is always and forever the sadness that we missed out on all these firsts with the baby we lost. And, more painfully, *they* missed out on them. To relieve a little of this heartbreak, you can dedicate the pride and happiness of your rainbow's milestone moments to the baby you lost. Whether it is in the instant it is happening, or in the time you spend reflecting afterwards, you can hold your lost baby tightly in your heart and think, *I'm thanking you, I'm dedicating this warm feeling to you, the accomplishments of my rainbow are a continuation of your lasting legacy.*

There is also the difficulty of explaining our new-found motherhood feelings to loved ones. While *we* may fully know that a rainbow baby is not ever a replacement for a baby we have lost and they are simply a joyful addition to our family, people around us may misunderstand that. They feel as though we have found what we were seeking, that now we have reached the end goal of 'a living baby' we are healed and can begin to move on. But loss mothers know that there is no such thing as moving on; closure is a concept that we do not believe in, nor do we really invite.

We have to open the conversation and tell those around us that we do not ever want to move on from our lost babies, because moving on means leaving them behind – and who wants to leave their children behind? When you are expected to be wholly joyful, there are moments where it can feel as though you are party pooping and forcibly dragging a black cloud over a happy occasion. You may feel as though you have already inflicted enough pain on those around you as you dealt with your previous loss and the need for their support through your early grief. You are left imagining that everyone is breathing a sigh of relief that you are now happy again. *Finally, a happy ending. Finally, an end to the sadness.* It comes with a new-found inner pressure to be simply happy and look to the future.

But while we are undoubtedly thrilled to have a baby in our arms, there is still equally a baby missing from them. Among the celebration of new life we are still mourning an all too early death. We know all too well that no matter how many babies we have there will always be one missing. To help those around us understand this we can share with them the definition of a rainbow baby. Perhaps we could ask them – with gentle grace – to put themselves in our shoes. If one of their children was to vanish, would a new baby's arrival erase the pain? We don't need to ask with confrontation, but as a way of offering fresh perspective. We can remind those around us that a baby is a child. It matters not how brief their life, we will love and miss them forever regardless of how our family grows.

A rainbow baby is an addition not a replacement.

There is a commonly shared feeling among loss mothers that having a rainbow baby is temporary. We cannot let ourselves believe that we will get to keep this new baby forever. Just as we expected the pregnancy to end at any point, we have now made it to birthing a living baby and still that feeling of impermanence lingers. It is as though we are waiting for our fears to be confirmed, living on a constant timer and one day soon that time will inevitably run out and we too will be separated. Always rumblings of, *What if ...,* and that nagging voice of, *Don't get too used to this, you know what can happen* ... It is so incredibly difficult to shake such fears and accept that, yes, you have a baby to love and to keep.

We feel that expecting the worst is a self-protection, that it is somehow necessary. It is something that humans are very good at doing – a belief that by waiting for bad news it will somehow soften the blow when it comes. But, actually, constantly expecting the worst just robs us of our happy present. As a bereaved mother, I fully understand that there is no switch to flick that will suddenly erase our deep-rooted fears. I have struggled immensely with post-loss anxiety and it is only to be expected following such a trauma. Whether you lost your previous baby through miscarriage, stillbirth or neonatal loss, your eyes have been opened to the fact that new life can end incredibly quickly and without warning. In these moments you have to trust your more rational mind, the mind that knows this is simply part of the deeply engrained world of life after loss. On that more rational level we know it is just emotional debris inflicted by a traumatic event and that our mind is untamed by grief. All new parents experience heightened awareness of their baby's well-being and as bereaved parents we are particularly delicate about the safety and wellness of our rainbow. But what we have here is a different baby with a different future and a different story to tell.

At times we may feel that by having the great gift of a rainbow baby in our arms – one that we have wanted so deeply and for so long – we are denied the chance to voice any natural struggles that come with mothering a living baby. There is a temptation to fall into the mindset of denying help or forcing ourselves to 'enjoy every single moment'. Finally we have what we want and it would wrong of us to complain or find it difficult. And so loss mothers can be particularly hard on themselves when faced with what are expected and universal challenges.

We know the true worth of a living baby, we are beyond grateful for the gift that lies in our arms, but learning how to care for a newborn baby is a giant learning curve for all mothers, *whether experienced in loss or not. It is OK to say 'I'm tired!' because babies are exhausting. It is OK to say 'I'm overwhelmed!' because babies require a whole new skillset and there is no definitive instruction book. It is OK to say 'I'm finding this hard!' because motherhood IS hard.*

It is hard regardless of previous loss, but particularly so when the pressure to never complain or seek help feels so high. Losing a baby certainly teaches us the true value of holding a living one, but it does not make you immune to the real challenges you face in learning to meet the constant and ever-changing needs of a tiny human. Allow yourself to reach out when you need it, guilt-free.

Your lost baby is not only an intrinsic part of your journey that brought you to this very day, but also a fundamental part of your rainbow baby's very existence. While everyone has their own ideas of life after death, I really do find comfort in imagining that my son had something to do with gifting us our daughter, and actually it's not such a far out truth. Had my son lived, had I not miscarried twice, would this exact version of my daughter exist here in my arms? Of course the ideal would involve all of our babies here with us, but the ideal will sadly never be a reality. What we can do is thank all our babies, no matter how swift their life.

As regrettable as the circumstances are, your previous baby's death created this new life. Their existence kick-started the cause and conditions for this new existence. Whether we had countless eggs sat in our ovaries ready to go or a limited edition carefully selected and waiting their turn, their opportunity to flourish into a fully fledged rainbow began in the hands of the baby we did not get to keep. Our lost baby had to exist in order for our rainbow to have their chance. In this sense we can see our rainbow as a gift, presented to us by our supremely kind lost baby. Your rainbow is a mastery of their creation.

Your lost baby may not have had a chance at life, they may have left without even an official meeting, but their life was never in vain. Among the many great lessons they taught us, they also left us a magnificent parting gift, a living baby in our arms.

With your lost baby in your heart and your rainbow in your arms, you can:

❋ Allow yourself to continue your grief. Even with new life you are still hurting for the baby you lost.
❋ Allow yourself to celebrate, too – your rainbow is a gift to be enjoyed.
❋ Expect that your grief may feel heightened at the new arrival, but trust that you will find your way once more.

✻ Look at ways to include both your babies in daily life and during celebrations.

✻ Know that you are still allowed to find your new version of motherhood difficult. Mothering a living baby is never easy or without challenges, regardless of any previous loss.

✻ Tell those close to you the meaning of a rainbow and explain that among the celebration you are still grieving your loss.

A LEGACY THAT LIVES ON

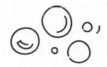

And so here you are, facing a lifetime ahead of you
without your most precious treasure. The very idea feels
overwhelming, bleak, an impossible mountain to climb. Even
with the possibility of a rainbow in our arms, there is the
never-ending torrent of pain that resides within baby loss.
We know that we will forever be missing a part of us, a face
always missing from photographs, an empty seat always
at the table, a shadow always absent from the sun. And as
bereaved parents we also know that happiness exists among
the heartbreak. Happy and sad, the two are not mutually
exclusive, instead they sit together like an old married couple,
sometimes residing peacefully and other times fighting to
stay together. We have stepped into this new world and there
is no option to step back out; this is our life now, happy/sad,
and we can embrace it with our baby always at the forefront
of our mind. Whether you choose to keep them privately
in your heart or share them with the world, how they are
remembered and celebrated rests on your shoulders.

From here on, your child's legacy is in your hands, you are the keepers of their destiny.

You can share their memory with friends and family, you can line the walls of your house with photographs or memories, you can write their names on Christmas cards, you can remember and mark the date you discovered their existence, and you can always include them on your journey forward.

And there are many things you can do practically, too. You may decide to become proactive within the baby loss community, either by raising money and supporting charities in memory of your baby or by raising the profile of loss within the healthcare industry.

You are your baby's voice. Whether you choose to use this voice as a gentle memorial whisper within your own private circle or as a vivid roar within the wider world, you can speak where your baby cannot. If you choose to dive into the wider loss community, you will find a wealth of love, support and encouragement. From your baby's life you can form new relationships and lifelong friendships within a network of fellow bereaved families that *really get* it. The baby loss club may not be a club that we had longed to become a part of, but once we are in it we find some of the most caring and uplifting families. It's a safe place to talk and share our babies, free from judgement, with people who inspire us to continue our baby's story.

Perhaps you will make a firm decision to support a charity that investigates the cause of miscarriage or SIDS

(Sudden Infant Death Syndrome), or you could gather together donations of premature babygrows to hand out at your local neonatal unit. Maybe you decide your local area is missing a memorial garden where you can remember your baby, and you bravely decide to put plans in place to create one. You could begin a blog and write about your loss, sharing experiences and helping others to understand, or you could simply dedicate some time to your baby's memory within your close family.

Like many who lose a child, Dean and I chose to focus our energy and love on the doctors and nurses who strived to save his life and raise the profile of the all-too-common tragedy of baby death. We began fundraising, and over time we raised enough to buy our local hospital a ventilator. The pride that comes with this is second to none – to know that our son's death may help another baby to live is a strange juxtaposition to sit with, but also happily peaceful. His life was so short he had so little time to make an impact on this big world, and yet here he is now giving the gift of life to many other poorly babies. With this act, our son has achieved more from his life than many who live into a ripe old age.

Sometimes you may feel as though it is exhausting, living in a constant state of fear that your baby will be forgotten. I don't know if that fear ever leaves us; I know it is still one of my greatest personal fears. While living babies grow into children and their physical presence and change is wide open for all to see, we are left with the trickier job of continually keeping our 'invisible' baby present. It can feel like a battle, and as though we are always having to remind the world of a life long gone. But you can do it. With your baby forever in your heart, you can speak their name and carry them into your future, including them in celebrations and life events.

We can remind people around us that our baby is ours always, not just for the moment they lived. And if anyone is busy thinking that this is odd, well, you can lend them this book, and you can trust that the face of baby loss is changing over time. One day – with a little help from all of us – all bereaved parents will be naturally expected to grieve and celebrate their babies forever. Our very own baby is part of this collective movement. You can shout their name or whisper it, share them publicly or hold them privately, whatever you choose to do you are including them in this magnificent transformation of the world's understanding of baby loss.

As our life continues and changes, so do our rituals. I used to visit my son's memorial every single Sunday without fail, with flowers in arms. Every monthly anniversary of his death would be spent reliving his life and death. A few years and a rainbow baby down the line and my life is different. Trips to his memorial are not so easy, sometimes his dates have passed me by without much notice. It's easy to beat yourself up and accuse yourself of forgetting. But we don't forget, we never forget. Just as life would evolve with our babies here, so it evolves without them.

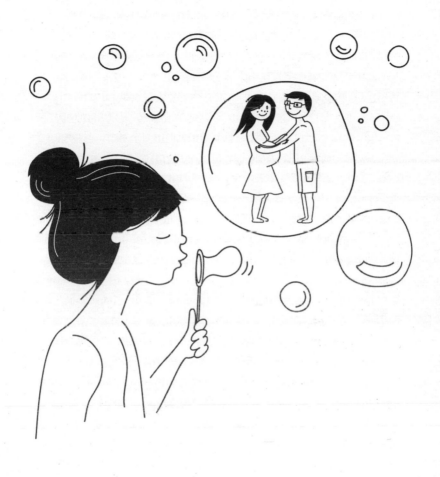

In those early throes of grief I would never imagine it possible, but life has a tendency to grow and change with us. It doesn't mean we won't still have our days of sitting on the bathroom floor and crying, or a week where we visit their memorial every single day as we are led by a sudden instinctive pull. But what I want to say is, it's OK if you loosen our desperate grip on the ceremonies that kept you going in those earlier days. You are not in the same place you were then, and while physical acts bring comfort they are ultimately not a defining measure of your love. As time goes on, your baby is simply acknowledged and celebrated in different, greater ways.

It is important to always remember to be kind to yourself, to trust your motherly instincts, to believe that however you continue to grieve your baby, it is the *right way* to grieve them for *you*. You can allow yourself the difficult days without judgement and the easier days without guilt. We know that our grief is everlasting, even if those around us do not. We can rest safe in the knowledge that all grieving parents the world over are understanding of this truth, and when we feel brave we can gently educate and share this understanding.

The path of life after baby loss is paved with uncertainty, and knowing this can leave us feeling lost and fragile. We rise, we plummet, we rise, we plummet. I have plummeted myself, dragging out my baby's memory box while soaked in tears, fraught over the dimming of my precious memories and my heart shattered as my son's smell fades from his single baby grow. It is true, there is no pain like that of a bereaved parent.

And just as you can trust that the dark days will come,
you can trust that they will live alongside the brighter days.

All lives are important, all lives have purpose, and
that includes even the lives that graced the earth so very
delicately.

From this point onwards you are a continuation of
their story. Your baby is trusting in you to lead the life they
were cheated out of, to be gentle and peaceful and leave a
positive, fitting mark on the world powerful enough for two
people. Our baby did not have the privilege of a life, but we
do. To waste it festering in hate and anger would be as if we
were saying 'It doesn't matter that you died, look, life is not
worth living anyway'. But of course it *does* matter because
life is worth living and it is worth celebrating, and there are
countless opportunities laid out for us to vividly include *all*
our children – whether that is adventuring up a mountain
and shouting your baby's name from the peak, or simply
a moment spent gathered with family and dedicating that
warm feeling to your baby – after all it was them who taught
us the importance of holding those we love so close.

You are their eyes and their feet. Wherever you go, they
go. They are made from you and so they are part of you. Did
you know that foetal cells circulate in a mother's blood? Once
you begin to grow your baby, their cells slipped into your body

and influenced your very DNA. That's real, that's science, that is your baby changing your very physicality and living on, quite literally, in you – in your blood, in your brain and in your heart. They have transformed you, they have taken up home inside your human body and eternally reshaped you.

And your baby's impact is never ending, they have altered you not only physically but also emotionally. While we inevitably continue to feel the pain inflicted by their death, we can also feel the love gifted by their life. Through the trauma and pain we shed our old skin like a slippery snake and emerge as a forever changed person. Battered and bruised yes, but also with a new sense of what our time on this earth is all about, a new understanding of grief and a new realisation of the fragility of life. With great thanks to your baby, you now truly see that life is fleeting and unpromised. You know that all meetings must end in partings and we must love each other while we have the chance.

Now our own hearts have been opened so wide, we see so easily the pain and suffering of those around us. Our babies taught us a new-found deep compassion and patience and we realise that amid all the ugliness in this world, there is boundless unbreakable love.

We can thank our babies for the biggest gift of all; the knowledge that love outlives even death.

HOW TO BE A
GOOD FRIEND

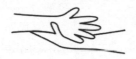

As you try to find your feet in this new world of loss, you will inevitably look around to your friends and family for support and comfort. Sometimes it can feel impossible to communicate our needs clearly, particularly in the early days or when our grief is especially choking, and those around us struggle to know what to say. This chapter is written with the idea that it can be shared with those you look to turn to, offering guidance and confidence in the support they can offer.

A loved one has experienced a huge loss. What do you do? How can you help? How do you ensure you bring comfort rather than add to the burden? Well,

You can be brave. You can gather courage in your belly and R E A C H O U T. Don't send the half-hearted text fluffed with well wishes of 'Call me if you need me'; understand that your friend can't always find the strength to pick up the phone. She doesn't want to be a burden, she doesn't want to ruin your day with misery and tears. Yes, her silence might be an indication of her need for space, but as a friend it is your duty to find out.

You can say 'I can't imagine your pain' rather than 'I know how you feel'.

You can say 'I don't know why this had to happen' rather than 'Everything happens for a reason'.

You can understand that some phrases that are banded about are not actually of any comfort at all. Her baby is not 'in a better place'; what better place is there than in a mother's arms? It is easy to say 'God needed another angel' when he didn't choose your own baby. You can refrain from saying 'at least' – 'at least you have other children', 'at least you know you can get pregnant', 'at least you didn't have to give birth', 'at least they lived for a while', 'at least you saw their eyes' … There is no *at least* when your baby has died. There are things to be celebrated yes, but nothing is ever compensation for the loss.

You can take the time to put yourself in your friend's shoes, as best as you can, and imagine what you would want to hear, what you would *really* want hear, not just repeat an outdated and miscalculated script. If you don't know what to say then say exactly that: 'I'm so sorry, I don't know what to say.'

You can open your ears. You can listen if your friend wants to talk about her baby, and listen if she doesn't. You can anticipate that some days she may want to sit within her own bubble and other days she may be seeking the courage to step out of it. You can hear the same story and the same emotions on repeat and listen as though it was the first time you have ever heard them.

If your friend wants to talk about her baby, then you can ask her about her baby. You can ask how it felt to hold them; did they look like her mum or her dad, did they have any little quirks like long fingers or big feet, did they have any hair, what colour was it? You can look at the bump photographs and see two people, a mother and a baby, and you can understand that life began long before birth. You can look at the grainy scan picture and realise that this was the beginnings of a little beating life, no matter how tiny and blurred to the eye – this was your friend's future. You can look at photographs of her baby without wincing. Photos of babies born prematurely, of those that have been stillborn or taken after a baby has died, may not look like the catalogue images we have been conditioned to see. You may notice the delicate pink paper-thin skin, the watercolours of bruising or the darkened lips, and these photographs may crush your heart, quite rightly so. But you can also see the loved baby, the wanted baby, the family photograph. You can shed a tear instead of a gasp, you can smile and comment, 'How beautiful your baby is!' You can be assured that all babies are beautiful whether dead or alive.

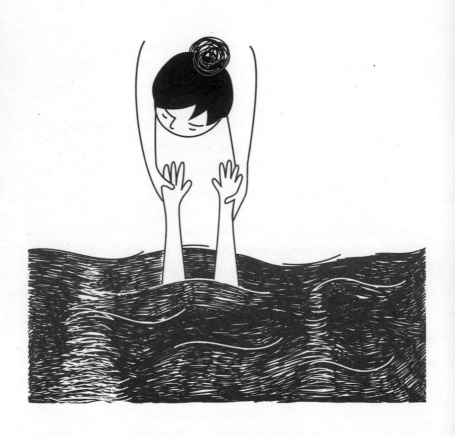

You can respect their grief. You can expect there will be days when she is happy and seemingly carefree, just as there will be days when she is glued to her duvet and hurting beyond belief. You can understand that there may be no rhyme or reason to her flow of emotions that day, that even the smallest reminder could be either a trigger or a comfort. You can know that time *doesn't* always heal, there is no breaking through to the 'other side' of grief, there is no 'getting over' her loss. Like a shadow, her grief is with her always but just not always so visible. You can recognise that next year she will be hurting, and the year after that, and even in ten, twenty, thirty years' time her heart will remain fractured. You can refrain from judging her grief, from suggesting she is grieving for too long or too hard. While time passes and her loss may feel like a long time ago, for her it is every day. You can know that talking about her baby doesn't mean she is stuck in the past, it simply means she is carrying them with her into her future. Perhaps she will go on to have more children, but she will always be missing one.

You can let her *own* her pain. Have we experienced something similar? Perhaps our grandma died, our aunty or our cat. It's not the same. It's never the same. Losing your baby is out of the natural order of life, burying a child isn't what we expect, not something we should have to do. Losing your baby is an experience within itself, there's no comparison to be made. We can draw from our personal experiences, yes, but we cannot compare. You can know that losing her baby is painful for *her* and that pain is *hers* to own.

You can be patient. You can know that grief is relentless and ongoing. You can understand that you may not always understand. You can trust that your friend is finding her way, in her own way, and that will take time. You can share the highs, catch the lows. You can know that a day of smiling and fundraising and inspirational thoughts can coexist alongside shattered grief and desperation to hold her baby.

It doesn't have to be one or the other, strong and weak, happy and sad, brave and fearful, they can all live beside each other. You can understand that they are irrevocably changed and yet still the same person we have always loved. You can recognise that her life will now and forever exist as a before and after, that she is no longer the person she once was. In the triumphs of the highs and the devastation of the lows, a whole new person has risen, an entirely altered life perspective and a whole new set of insecurities and doubt.

You can see that despite this monumental shift, your friend is still your friend. Different but the same. Still human, still doing daily chores and still laughing at your long-standing jokes, but now a little bruised around the heart, cancelling some plans because she's tired, *truly tired*, and hibernating when the celebrations that roll around feel impossible.

You can join in her remembrance. You can celebrate her baby alongside her. You can tell her when you have been thinking about her baby, send a message as you pass by the butterfly or the snowflake or the flower that sparks their legacy. You can carry them with you on trips and holidays, write their names in the sand on your beach walk, and light a candle in their memory at the historical cathedral. You can remind her that her baby is never forgotten and is loved far and wide. You can speak her baby's name with confidence and love. Never are we reminding her that her baby died, she will never forget that, instead you remind her that they lived, they are loved and they are remembered.

You can give them the gift of T I M E. Great big slices of our lifetime boxed up with a huge generous bow. Time together, time apart, time remembering, time talking, time listening, time doing, time being. Lashings of time, carefully considered and gently distributed. You can keep the silent promise you made in your friendship to just *be there*. Whether you are putting together a food parcel in those dark days when eating is a chore, or smiling as your friend recalls the moment she first discovered she was pregnant. Physically, virtually, emotionally. You can be there.

And finally, the greatest gift you can give to a bereaved mother is the knowledge that her baby will be forever remembered. Whether your friend publicly shares her baby or keeps her loss so very private and close to her heart, you can bet your bottom dollar she is fearful her baby will be forgotten. You can follow her lead and include her baby in life events. Address a Christmas card to mother, father *and* baby. If that feels too bold then add 'and remembering baby'. A mother and father N E V E R forget their baby, can you ever imagine forgetting your own?

Living or not, once they are created their existence is forever. You can give your friend the greatest gift by simply remembering her baby.

HELP
& SUPPORT

Tommy's

Funds research into miscarriage, stillbirth and premature birth, and provides pregnancy health information to parents.

www.tommys.org

Sands

Stillbirth and neonatal death charity supporting anyone affected by the death of a baby, working to improve the care bereaved parents receive, and promoting research to reduce the loss of babies' lives.

www.sands.org.uk

Aching Arms

A baby loss charity run by a group of bereaved mothers whose aim is to raise awareness of the impact of pregnancy and baby loss and bring some comfort to bereaved parents and their families.

www.achingarms.co.uk

Kicks Count
An app that lets you get to know your baby's regular pattern
of movement.

www.kickscount.org.uk

Miscarriage Association
Information and support for those affected by miscarriage,
molar pregnancy or ectopic pregnancy.

www.miscarriageassociation.org.uk

Pregnancy After Loss Support (PALS)
A community loss support resource for women experiencing
the confusing and conflicting emotions of grief mixed with joy
during the journey through pregnancy after loss.

www.pregnancyafterlosssupport.com

Saying Goodbye
Provides comprehensive information, advice, support and
much more to anyone who has suffered the loss of a baby, at
any stage of pregnancy, at birth or in infancy.

www.sayinggoodbye.org

Tharpa Publications
Buddhist resources for further information on ways to
understand our mind, manage our negative emotions and
harvest compassion in our day-to-day lives.

www.tharpa.com/uk

On Instagram and Twitter, the hashtags #babyloss, #miscarriage and #ttc will connect you to a whole world of loss mothers.

ACKNOWLEDGEMENTS

Writing this book was quite literally a labour of love, and it simply would not have been possible without the incredible support network I have around me. I would like to thank with a full heart my husband Dean, for putting up with my absolute inept ability to focus beyond the book and the baby, for feeding me, watering me and keeping me calm, and above all for being co-creator of our beautiful children.

Thank you to my mum for looking after Raven at the drop of a hat and taking holidays from work to help with my workload. And to the rest of my amazing family and friends for their endless encouragement, providing snacks and mental refuge, their kind words of support and their continuing remembrance of Winter.

Thank you to all the sangha at Tara Kadampa Meditation Centre for opening my eyes to new ways of thinking and helping me to turn my immense loss into something beautiful, proactive and meaningful.

Thank you to anyone and everyone that I have met along this journey – all the families, every single mother with or without her baby. By offering your insights and sharing your gorgeous babies with me you have given me extra energy to write this book.

Acknowledgements

Thank you to Clemmie Telford for passing on my details to Sam Jackson, my publisher, and therefore helping this book to come into fruition. Thank you to Farrah Moore and Michelle Cottle for reading my manuscript and offering guidance from other loss perspectives. Thank you Nora Leinad for providing the beautiful illustrations to accompany my writing.

And thank you to the team at Vermilion for inviting this opportunity into my life, particularly Sam for her remarkable patience and guidance. For so long I had wanted to write a book about baby loss and you guys made a dream a reality.

Thank you Winter for being an absolute inspiration in my life now and forever, and thank you Raven for not only being a total dream but for arriving at exactly the right time to enable me to write this book!

ABOUT THE AUTHOR

Nicola – affectionately known as Pea – is a tiny human with colourful hair and a keen interest in Buddhism. Having travelled to over 30 countries together, she finally married Dean in a secret beach wedding in Sri Lanka. This is her first ever book, written as her daughter napped and nursed.

Nicola's first baby, a son named Winter Wolfe, was born with dark brown eyes and lips that naturally rested in a smile. Shortly after his delivery Winter became suddenly unwell and sadly he died the next day, held peacefully in the arms of his parents. His life was swift but not without love, and Nicola, having publicly shared her pregnancy, made the decision to continue writing about her little boy, the grief she experienced, her journey of trying to conceive after loss, her subsequent miscarriages and the arrival of her daughter Raven Rain.

Instagram @onedayofwinter
Blog www.onedayofwinter.com
YouTube onedayofwinter
Twitter @_onedayofwinter

1 3 5 7 9 10 8 6 4 2

Vermilion, an imprint of Ebury Publishing,
20 Vauxhall Bridge Road,
London SW1V 2SA

Vermilion is part of the Penguin Random House group of companies
whose addresses can be found at global.penguinrandomhouse.com

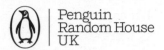
Penguin
Random House
UK

Published in the United Kingdom by Vermilion in 2018

www.penguin.co.uk

A CIP catalogue record for this book is available
from the British Library

ISBN 9781785042027

Typeset in 9/15.2 pt Caecilia LT Std
by Integra Software Services Pvt. Ltd, Pondicherry

Printed and bound in Great Britain by Clays Ltd, Elcograf S.p.A.

Penguin Random House is committed to a sustainable future
for our business, our readers and our planet. This book is
made from Forest Stewardship Council® certified paper.

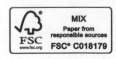
MIX
Paper from
responsible sources
FSC® C018179